The Pelvic Floor Bible

Jane Simpson has had her own private practice for twenty-two years where she treats patients with all forms of incontinence and pelvic floor dysfunction. She is a member of the Pelvic Floor Society, the Association for Continence Advice and the International Continence Society. This is her first book, which she hopes will spread the word on a global scale that pelvic floor dysfunction is curable and does not need to be life-changing or limiting.

THE PELVIC FLOOR BIBLE

*Everything You Need to Know to Prevent and Cure
Problems at Every Stage of Your Life*

JANE SIMPSON

PENGUIN LIFE

AN IMPRINT OF

PENGUIN BOOKS

PENGUIN LIFE

UK | USA | Canada | Ireland | Australia
India | New Zealand | South Africa

Penguin Life is part of the Penguin Random House group of companies
whose addresses can be found at global.penguinrandomhouse.com.

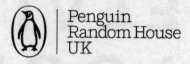

Penguin
Random House
UK

First published 2019
001

Diagrams by Rachael Tremlett

The questionnaire on pages 114–15 is from 'Development and evaluation of
an abridged, 5-item version of the International Index of Erectile Function
(IIEF-5) as a diagnostic tool for erectile dysfunction' by R. C. Rosen, J. C.
Cappelleri and M. D. Smith, and has been reproduced by kind permission
of *IJIR: Your Journal of Sexual Medicine*; and the stool chart on page 125 is
from 'Vesicoureteral reflux – the role of bladder and bowel dysfunction'
by Jack S. Elder and Mireya Diaz, and has been reproduced by kind
permission of *Nature Reviews Urology*

Set in 9/12.75 pt ITC Stone Serif Std
Typeset by Jouve (UK), Milton Keynes
Printed and bound in Great Britain by Clays Ltd, Elcograf S.p.A.

A CIP catalogue record for this book is available from the British Library

ISBN: 978–0–241–38653–8

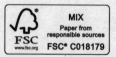

For William and Charles, with love

CONTENTS

LIST OF ILLUSTRATIONS

Chapter 9

Chapter 10

INTRODUCTION

We should all be doing pelvic floor exercises – and I mean everyone: young and old, male and female, wherever you live in the world. It's an absolutely vital part of our physical wellbeing, is incredibly easy and, as you'll see throughout this book, can be utterly life-changing. I hope what you read in the pages that follow not only answers all your questions about your pelvic floor but empowers you to change the way you think and to start to care about your pelvic floor the same way that you care about the rest of your body.

Pelvic floor dysfunction commonly occurs in women either after having a baby or during the menopause. However, it affects men too and is commonly associated with prostate problems. What is less known is that it can happen to us at any time in our life and sometimes totally out of the blue, so be prepared to start working on your muscle training straight away! Don't think you're immune from danger if you haven't or aren't planning to give birth. A recent review concluded that sports practice increases the prevalence of urinary incontinence, with high-impact sports causing the most incontinence.[1] Another review concluded that training the pelvic floor muscles can cure or improve symptoms of stress urinary incontinence and all other types of incontinence.[2] So you have the proof that now is the time to get started!

It's never too late to start pelvic floor rehabilitation, so I don't want anyone thinking, what's the point, I am beyond help. That's never the case! As we are all living longer and are much more active in our later years it's even more vital that we maintain healthy bodies, and that includes your pelvic floor muscles. If you are young then please don't think that this doesn't concern you – think of what all that high-impact exercise you enjoy so much is doing to you. Pelvic floor exercises, when done correctly, take up just a few moments of your day and should be part of your normal routine, regardless of whether you've suffered any problems thus far, so it's important to get into the habit – much like brushing your teeth.

If you are suffering from problems – and perhaps these are issues you've struggled with for years – then I hope this book will open up the discussion and break the taboo once and for all. Why should it be embarrassing? These are all too common problems that should be discussed openly. There is so much advice and support out there so let my book guide you and show you how to help yourself and, if necessary, where to find the right people or organizations to help you.

I started my general nurse's training in 1980 at Addenbrooke's Hospital in Cambridge and went on to become a district nursing sister. This is where my interest in incontinence and pelvic floor dysfunction started, as every day I was seeing people suffering the indignity of urinary or faecal incontinence, reduced to wearing incontinence pads that were – at that time – one size fits all. This made me realize that there had to be something better. In the early 1990s I became a continence nurse specialist in the NHS when the specialism was just starting to grow. I am still a continence specialist at the London Clinic, where I have had the privilege of working with world-renowned gynaecologists, urologists, colorectal surgeons, gastroenterologists and many other doctors from all specialities. I have now been treating people with pelvic floor dysfunction for more than twenty-five years and I have enjoyed every minute of it. I have thousands of stories; I'd like to share a couple that sum up my reasons for finally writing this book, because it's clear that there are so many ill-founded myths about what people can do to take charge of problems.

I had a patient several years ago who was referred to me for treatment by her gynaecologist. When we first met she was extremely sceptical about pelvic floor rehabilitation and had assumed that she would need an operation. At the end of her treatment, completely cured of all of her problems, with no surgical intervention whatsoever, she reminded me of our first encounter and with a wry smile said, 'It's a good job I didn't have an operation – look at me now! Problem solved.'

Another patient of mine was thirty-five years old, she had not had any children and had been suffering with urge incontinence for five years. She may well still be suffering if it hadn't been for her mother, whom I had also treated for stress incontinence. She told me how worried she was about her daughter; she had stopped going out, was very down and was talking about leaving her job. She had no idea what was the matter with her. Her mother did really well with her pelvic floor rehabilitation and then about three months later her daughter came to see me out of the blue. She had confided in her mother about the awful urinary frequency and urgency and, worse, the urge incontinence that she had. As a result she had retreated into her shell and may well have stayed there if it wasn't for her mother seeking help for her own condition. She is now completely better. These are the encounters that give me joy every time.

I hope this book makes you smile – and sometimes squirm – in places and in others say, 'I know, I know, that's me.' Most importantly, I hope it motivates you to take the time to focus on your pelvic floor and live a happier and more carefree life as a result. Never suffer in silence again – it's time to start a pelvic floor revolution.

PART ONE

The Fundamentals

ONE

What is the Pelvic Floor? Understanding Your Anatomy

Your pelvic floor is made up of a group of muscles that stretch from your tailbone (coccyx) at the back to your pubic bone at the front and between the bones that you sit on, from one side to the other. These muscles work a bit like a piece of elastic or a trampoline. They have the ability to move up and down as needed, depending on what you are doing. There are gaps in the pelvic floor especially designed to allow the urethra, vagina and anus to pass through.

Your pelvic floor muscles are just that – the floor of your pelvic cavity, acting like a hammock to provide the main support for your pelvic organs. Without them your internal abdominal and pelvic organs would simply fall out! Your pelvic floor muscles are wrapped tightly around the urethra, vagina and anus in women, and around the urethra and anus in men. They are able to contract when you cough or sneeze to help keep you continent and prevent you from leaking.

However, with your conscious control they allow you to decide when to pass urine or open your bowels (and make sure that you don't fart at an awkward moment!). In pregnant women, the pelvic floor cradles your baby as it grows bigger and also helps you when you are giving birth. In addition, the pelvic floor plays a

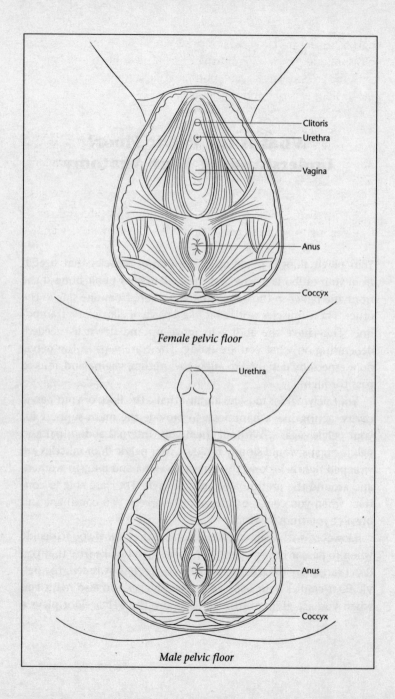

Female pelvic floor

Male pelvic floor

part in sexual function for both sexes, helping to increase sexual pleasure and contracting during orgasm in women, and helping with the erection and ejaculation function in men. So really, your pelvic floor is very important indeed!

The Pelvic Floor Muscles
Your pelvic floor muscles are made up of two types of muscle fibres. The fibres are important and each one has an individual role.

- Slow twitch muscle fibres – these are responsible for the resting tone of the pelvic floor. They are slow to tire and help to keep us continent.
- Fast twitch muscle fibres – we have far fewer fast twitch fibres; they work when a quick powerful contraction is needed, for example when you cough or sneeze.

The Bony Bits
Your pelvis, bony pelvis or your pelvic girdle is largely made up of your hip bones at the sides and front and your sacrum and coccyx (the last bit of your spine) at the back. Your hip bones are attached to your sacrum at the back and to each other at the front where they meet the symphysis pubis joint. Both of your legs and your spine (backbone) are attached to your pelvis: your legs left and right at either side and your spine at the back. The hole through the middle of your pelvis is called the pelvic cavity and it is here that your pelvic floor is located.

Your Core
Your pelvic floor is part of what we call our core; in fact, it is the bottom of your core. At the front you have your abdominal muscles, at the back your mid to lower back muscles and on top your respiratory diaphragm; together all these parts make up our core. Your core works together to support your spine, keep you

standing upright and give you stability. It helps with your posture and with your movement and mobility.

The Anus and Anal Sphincters
Your anus is the last part of your gastrointestinal tract and is the external opening at the end of the rectum. Your anus is the bit that passes through your pelvic floor muscles.

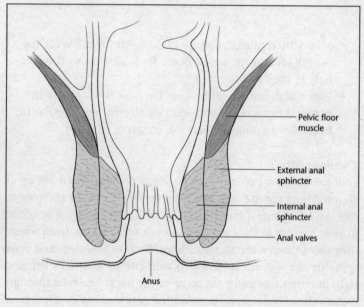

Anus and anal sphincters

Your anal sphincters are wrapped around your anus and are what control defecation, allowing us to control when we poo. There are two muscles, the internal anal sphincter and the external anal sphincter. They work together to signal to you when you need to go to the toilet – and whether it's an emergency or not! Your external anal sphincter is the one you have the ability to contract and relax and have conscious control over. Together the two muscles signal to your brain whether you need a poo, are going to have diarrhoea or if you need to pass wind. When they work together properly they allow you to control when you do all of these things.

Your rectum works as a storage chamber until you can find a toilet; at that point you can relax your anal sphincters to open your bowels. Once you have finished, the anal sphincters contract again to keep you continent.

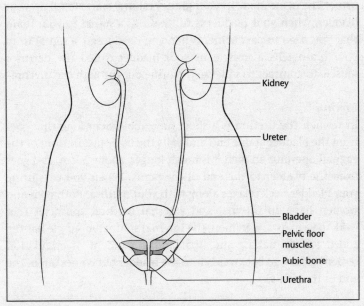

Your urinary system is made up of your kidneys, ureters, bladder and urethra, all of which work together closely.

Kidneys

Urine is produced in your kidneys, which are located at the bottom of your ribcage, one on either side of your spine; they are about the size of your fist or a computer mouse. They work by filtering your blood to remove waste and any extra fluid that your body doesn't need. This waste is turned into urine.

Ureters

Your urine then passes down both your ureters, which are the tubes that connect each of your kidneys to your bladder.

Bladder

Your bladder is a storage bag, a bit like a balloon made of muscle that sits in the lower part of your abdomen. It is about the same size as a pear when empty and its purpose is to collect and store urine. The urine made in your kidneys slowly starts to fill up your bladder; when your bladder is full it sends a signal to your brain that you need to pass urine. When you need to go, a signal from your brain tells a muscle in your bladder called the detrusor muscle to contract to squeeze the urine out through the urethra.

Urethra

In women the urethra is a short tube about 5cm long that goes from the bladder at one end and exits the body just in front of the vaginal opening. In men it is much longer, about 20cm, and goes from the bladder to the end of the penis. When you pass urine your bladder neck relaxes along with your urethra. Both men and women have an internal and external urethral sphincter that work to keep us dry. In men, the internal sphincter muscle has the added job of making sure that at the moment of ejaculation semen doesn't go backwards into the bladder but comes out of the end of the penis.

Your pelvic floor muscles are (as are all muscles of the human body) pretty amazing but sadly they are much neglected; they are probably the most ignored muscles in our bodies, even when they are malfunctioning. I am sure that this is largely due to the fact that we can't see them or visualize them, unlike our abs that many of us are busily striving to make flat and perfectly toned. However, I suspect we all know that we have pelvic floor muscles, from clenching our anal sphincter in a bid to suppress a fart or squeezing our pelvic floor when fumbling with the key on the doorstep to prevent an emergency dash to the toilet.

The muscles, nerves, ligaments, connective tissue and blood vessels that work to help your pelvic floor function will not let you down if you do your pelvic floor exercises regularly. If you make them the norm, as you might with any other exercises that you seemingly 'must do', your body will always thank you.

TWO

The Ultimate Guide to Pelvic Floor Rehabilitation: Tools and Techniques to Build Pelvic Floor Strength

Pelvic floor rehabilitation has been around in some form for thousands of years. Hippocrates, Galen and others devised pelvic exercise regimens to be followed in the baths and gymnasia of ancient Greece and Rome as it was thought that strengthening this group of muscles would promote physical wellbeing and sexual health.

A very ancient manuscript from 1500 BC talks about managing urinary incontinence with pads. I wonder what they were made of? It's hard to believe that the millions of incontinence pads sold around the world every year have such an ancient origin.

Across different cultures the practice of contracting your pelvic floor muscles has historically been thought to have many different purposes. Chinese Taoists have practised pelvic floor exercises for over 6,000 years in the form of something called the Deer exercise; this involves circular rubbing of the breasts in women or the lower abdomen in men while contracting the perineum and holding/pulling up or squeezing your pelvic floor muscles for as long as possible, usually about a minute. They thought that this would increase sexual energy, health and spiritual wellbeing. Ancient Indian texts give details of similar exercises as part of the Ashwini Mudra, or gesture of the horse, part of a yoga technique that involves contracting your anal sphincter in a rhythmic way. It is thought to bring many physical, emotional and spiritual benefits such as toning pelvic muscles, improving sexual health and calming or boosting your mood.

Skipping forward a few centuries to 1936, Margaret Morris, a dancer, choreographer and trained physiotherapist in London, stressed the importance of core muscles and posture and wrote about maternity and post-operative exercises. She was ahead of her time in teaching women how to contract and relax their pelvic floor muscles.

In the 1940s Arnold Kegel, an American gynaecologist, noticed that following childbirth his patients' pelvic floor muscles were not working as well as they had done before pregnancy. I am sure other gynaecologists had reached the same conclusions but it was Arnold Kegel who decided to do something about it by inventing the Kegel perineometer. This was a soft probe attached to a

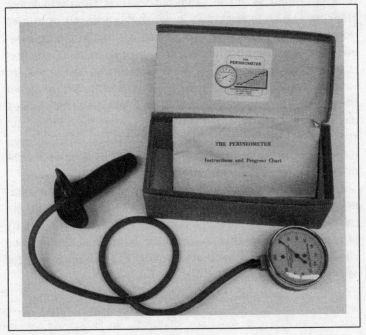

Kegel perineometer

pressure gauge (a bit like a car speedometer!) that a woman could insert into her vagina to give a reading when she contracted her pelvic floor muscles. This allowed his patients to measure their pelvic floor strength and, over time, track their progress to check that their strength was improving with rehabilitation. He then gave his patients a programme of pelvic floor exercises and a perineometer to take home so that they could do their exercises in the comfort of their own home and monitor their progress at the same time.

What a legacy to then have those exercises named after him. I hope that he would have a wry smile today reading this, knowing that we are trying to motivate a whole world full of women to do their exercises.

The Kegel perineometer was one of the first vaginal biofeedback machines; as anyone addicted to their Fitbit will know, allowing women to track their progress motivates them to keep doing the exercises regularly. It probably is worth noting, however, that Kegel set his patients a serious programme of exercises that were more suited to the 1940s housewife than to the modern working women of today. The daily regime involved carrying out the exercises with the perineometer for 20 minutes, three times a day![3] All the same, his ideas were revolutionary for his time and started something amazing. They are still being used today, even if they now are in the form of apps and other bits of modern technology that we're about to explore.

In this chapter we are going to look at pelvic floor rehabilitation in the form of exercises, which will make up part of the treatment in most of the chapters of this book. They are a big part of your recovery, whether your problem is stress incontinence or any one of the other issues that we will look at through the course of *The Pelvic Floor Bible*.

Pelvic Floor Exercises for Women

The most important thing about pelvic floor exercises is to isolate and use the right muscles, and then to make the exercises part of your everyday routine, not just when you see my book looking at you or you have the odd leak of urine. It has to become part of your daily life. It's so easy but so very important.

Follow the techniques described below to develop an awareness of your pelvic floor muscles. At first you might find it hard not to just squeeze your buttocks or your legs together; it's also important to breathe normally, so try not to hold your breath.

- Sit on the arm of a chair, an exercise or fitness ball or any hard surface with your feet flat on the floor. Lean slightly forward with your vulval area in contact with the hard surface. With your hands on your thighs try to lift the area around your vagina and anus away from whatever it is you are sitting on.
- If you are a tampon user, try inserting one, then pull gently on the string. At the same time contract your muscles around the tampon to stop it coming out, a bit like a tug of war. This is a good way of helping you to isolate and use the correct muscles.
- Sit up straight on the toilet with your knees apart. While passing urine, try to stop the flow by contracting your muscles up and inwards. Squeeze, lift and hold for a moment and then let go. Don't worry if the flow did not stop altogether but remember which set of muscles you used. This is just a test to figure out which muscles you are contracting so do not do this on a regular basis as it can be harmful to your bladder.
- When you are having sex try to squeeze your partner's penis. This may help you isolate your pelvic floor muscles.

You can also insert your finger into your vagina and see if you are able to squeeze it.

- Pretend you are controlling an attack of diarrhoea or about to pass wind. Pull up the muscles around your anus, squeeze, lift and hold. I often tell my patients to imagine that they are in a lift full of people and need to pass wind, what would they do?

These muscles you have been tightening are your pelvic floor muscles. They include the ones around your anus and the ones around your vagina. They form the cradle of muscles that support your rectum, vagina and urethra as detailed in Chapter 1. You should use all of these muscles together when performing the exercises.

If you are still not sure that you have isolated the correct muscles, please seek help. Most health authorities have specialist continence nurses and women's health physiotherapists who can help you to engage with the correct muscles.

HOW TO PERFORM YOUR PELVIC FLOOR EXERCISES

To start with it's probably better to do the exercises lying on your back with your feet flat on the floor and knees bent, or sitting on a chair or fitness ball, leaning slightly forward with your hands on your thighs (as if you were sitting on the toilet). You can do the exercises standing and I'm sure most of you have heard at one time or another that you can do your pelvic floor exercises 'while standing at the bus stop'; however, as gravity has a part to play when you are standing, and particularly if you have a prolapse, it makes sense to start off sitting or lying down.

1. Draw up all the muscles at the same time, squeeze, lift and hold for a count of five, if you can.
2. If you feel that your muscles have let go before you get to five just hold for as many seconds as you can. Keep practising and try to slowly build up until you can hold for ten seconds – this could take you a few weeks or even longer. You may have to start by contracting your muscles for just one second, and this is totally fine. The great news is that you have started and are on the road to recovery.
3. Once you have held on for up to ten seconds let go gently and count to five – this is the rest phase of the programme. It is very important not to overtire your muscles, particularly when you are just starting and your muscles are weak.
4. You then need to repeat the same exercise (hold for ten seconds and release for five seconds) five times. This will take a few minutes each day.
5. Try to do the exercises three times per day but don't worry if you occasionally only manage it once or twice a day – at least you are doing it. It has to work for you.

Once a day, you should also do a series of ten short, sharp contractions. These are done in a rhythmic pattern of squeeze, let go, squeeze, let go and will help you maintain control when you need to suddenly sneeze or cough.

It is likely to take several weeks before you start to see an improvement. Whatever you do, don't give up – please persevere and continue the exercises even after you start to notice an improvement.

You may find it more difficult to do the exercises in the evening, as your muscles tend to be tired like the rest of your body. It's also possible that you notice a mild aching sensation shortly after starting the exercise programme; this is usually due to your muscles becoming tired, just as they would with any form of fitness regime. Any pelvic floor muscle ache should subside as your muscles get stronger, but if the aching persists just stop doing the exercises for a couple of days.

The Knack
This 'knack' came about following a piece of research that found that a well-timed contraction of your pelvic floor muscles when you are about to cough or sneeze has the effect of helping you not to leak, at that exact moment. It was also found to protect your pelvic floor muscles, so it has a double benefit and is well worth trying to remember to do.

Core Strength
Our core is important for our posture, for the stability of our spine and for movement. Our core is made up from the pelvic floor muscles at the bottom, the abdominal and back muscles, and the respiratory diaphragm at the top. I'm sure lots of you have discovered 'core exercises' at the gym or in a class but if you have a weak pelvic floor or know that you have diastasis recti (see Chapter 6) you should be very careful not to do some core exercises like sit-ups or crunches. If in doubt ask a professional as striving for the perfect body may mean you damage your pelvic floor further.

Getting into the Habit
I firmly believe that a pelvic floor exercise programme should be very personal and tailored to your lifestyle. That way you are much more likely to do it than feel frustrated that you haven't managed the programme that you read about or that has been set for you. So make a plan and stick to it. I tell my patients to try to associate the exercises with something that they do every day. For example, when they are on the school run, watching the news, on the bus or train to work, or as simple as when they are cleaning

their teeth – we will all do that every day so why not your pelvic floor exercises? Once you are able to associate doing your pelvic floor exercises with performing daily tasks it will become a habit and much easier to remember. The most important thing is to establish a routine that you can follow on a daily basis.

I have always tried very hard to tailor treatment to maximize compliance. Most women are juggling lots of different priorities so pelvic floor rehabilitation is often a low priority. However, if the treatment is quick and easy to do, doesn't involve numerous trips to a clinic or time out of every day to perform a course of exercises, then I am very sure everyone's pelvic floor would be in a better shape.

If pelvic floor exercises are not for you, or maybe you have desperately been trying to contract you pelvic floor and not a lot seems to be happening, then please don't despair and whatever you do don't give up. In this next section you'll find information about the many tools and gadgets that can help you.

Tools and Gadgets

So many women have come to see me with some gadget or other and said, 'I bought this five years ago and have never got round to using it [like "it" is the elephant in the room] but my stress incontinence is now much worse. I really need to do something.' Does this ring a bell with you?

The Squeezy App for Women

There is a very good app called Squeezy. You can follow a pre-set exercise programme in the exercise plan section of the app, or you can tailor the app to a doable pelvic floor programme for yourself. It may be that your healthcare professional has set a programme for you. The app will even remind you to do your exercises, which in most cases is half the battle. I see women every week who tell me, 'I so want to do my exercises but I keep forgetting.' The app has the ability to time your pelvic floor contractions, so no cheating and counting to ten really fast! It also counts the rest phase of the exercise, which is also very important. It has a bladder diary setting that you do over three days, which may give you an insight into what is happening with your fluid intake and urine output, information that will be very helpful if you ever need to see a specialist healthcare professional. It also has lots of helpful tips about bladder health.

Vaginal Weights

I had a patient who loved this product so much that she bought one for each of her two daughters for Christmas. She wrapped them up and put them under the Christmas tree – you can only begin to imagine the amazement of her daughters when they opened their gifts on Christmas morning. That would certainly have been an unusual conversation to have over the turkey!

Vaginal weights, or vaginal cones, are a selection of small tampon-like objects in different sizes, shaped so that they can be comfortably held in the vagina. They vary in weight starting with the lightest cone being about 5 grams. You move up in weight incrementally as your muscles become stronger and you are able to hold heavier weights, the heaviest of which is usually between 50 and 70 grams. You may never manage to hold the heaviest weight and that doesn't matter at all; what matters is whether you are improving and if the answer is yes, then you have done really well, whatever the weight achieved. The cone is held in place by a natural reflex contraction of the pelvic floor; the action of the weighted cone in the vagina exercises the muscles. You need to start with the lightest weight and slowly increase it. They are a great way to improve vaginal muscles, are easy to use and not too expensive. You should use them when you are in the shower in the morning and while you are getting ready for the day, ideally for 10–20 minutes.

However, as a word of warning, don't forget to take the cone out before you leave the house. I have had many patients who have done just that, only to find themselves in the supermarket or the office, their muscles are tired and, you guessed it, a rather embarrassing moment happens!

The great thing about this type of therapy is it allows you to track how well you are doing and this helps you to monitor your progress. As you progress on to heavier weights you can see improvement – achieving positive results is so important.

However, this treatment is not for everyone, particularly women with prolapse, but if you have a busy life and mild stress incontinence, this is a good, easy way to start improving your pelvic floor tone.

Electrical Stimulation

Electrical stimulation is something that is either performed in a clinic by a pelvic floor specialist or using machines that are available to buy online (they can also be found in very specialized pharmacies or from healthcare professionals). There are several machines on the market with a variety of programmes. How do you know if electrical stimulation is for you? A good indication is if you feel you have no awareness of your pelvic floor contracting. If your antenatal or Pilates class teacher tells you to squeeze the pelvic floor, do you have a clue what to do? Can you try to stop the flow of urine midstream? Or, when you are having sex, are you able to squeeze your partner's penis? Maybe try inserting your finger into your vagina and seeing if you can squeeze it – can you feel your muscles contracting at all? If the answer to these questions is no, then electrical stimulation is for you. It's a great way to try to wake up your muscles.

The machines work by inserting a small electrode into the vagina. A low-voltage current stimulates the muscles, making them contract. You usually need to follow a programme that is 20–30 minutes long and many machines have various programmes so look for the ones specifically designed for pelvic floor strengthening. Start with the gentlest programme and then move on to more challenging ones when your muscles have started to work again. In general, you need to sit or lie down to do this so a certain level of commitment is required. Lots of my patients are delighted to have the excuse to lie down for half an hour in the middle of their busy lives – you could even catch up on your emails, watch TV or make a phone call as the machine does the work for you. If you have very weak pelvic floor muscles this is a great place to start. As with all things there are contraindications to using electrical stimulation devices: these include pregnancy, having an abnormal smear test result, having a pacemaker and while you are on your period. Always read the instructions before buying or using a machine and, if in any doubt at all, seek medical advice.

The good news is there are enough devices to suit everyone. It's wonderful to hear women who have been using a machine like this come back and say, 'I had forgotten what my vagina used to feel like!' Often sexual pleasure is improved as well, which is a fabulous bonus.

Elvie and Similar Devices

The next treatments are definitely for the modern woman and work with an app. They are small, intravaginal devices that connect wirelessly to your smartphone. They put you through a programme of exercises designed for all levels of pelvic floor strength – as you squeeze you can see the results in real time using biofeedback (see below), thanks to great graphics that show and track your progress, giving you instant feedback and guidance. I think the feedback element is extremely encouraging and very motivating; they also provide you with a viewable workout history. I even have a few patients who happen to be friends who compete with each other for the best score! Two of my patients who are friends have become so competitive that the one with the best score that week gets treated to lunch by the other one! I am just delighted that they are both using whatever means to motivate themselves to improve their pelvic floor health.

Although there are lots of gadgets and devices on the market, I have given you the main examples here. If you have bought something or been recommended something else by a healthcare professional or friend and it's working for you, that's great. I just want you to get better so if your symptoms are improving then that is good with me.

As you can imagine, doing pelvic floor exercises in conjunction with one of the treatments above will hopefully be very motivating – and motivation is the key! It's vital and makes logical sense: if you are using a gadget and seeing improvements, like holding heavier weights, or seeing visual improvements on the app, your motivation should stay high. However, this doesn't mean that doing your pelvic floor exercises alone isn't enough – it is. We are all different and all I am trying to do is make sure that everyone finds the right way forward. Ultimately we all want the same result – the perfect pelvic floor! I hope that what you take away from reading this chapter is the knowledge of how to do your pelvic floor exercises correctly and the inspiration to start.

Biofeedback

Biofeedback is used in lots of different therapies to gain better awareness of bodily functions. You can also say that when someone smiles and waves at you this is positive biofeedback that they are happy to see you.

For our purposes in pelvic floor muscle training, biofeedback simply means that when you contract your pelvic floor muscles you get a reaction. A way of doing this at home is to insert a finger into your vagina and see if you can squeeze it, then try a week later to see if you are able to squeeze your finger harder than the last time you tried. If you are using vaginal weights, being able to hold heavier vaginal weights is positive biofeedback. Maybe you are getting better scores with your Elvie. It is all about giving you the motivation to continue with whatever therapy you are doing by seeing some positive feedback.

Probably a more traditional form of biofeedback is performed in a clinic setting, where a vaginal or anal (for men) probe is inserted that is then connected to a biofeedback machine. At this point you will be asked to contract your pelvic floor muscles; you will then be able to see a graph showing how your muscles are working. I use this form of therapy with nearly all of my patients. It is very motivating to see accurate graphs monitoring your progress. Everyone's first words when they come in through the door are, 'I wonder what my score will be today, I have been working really hard on my exercises at home.' But we are also human so sometimes they will say, 'I know I haven't done so well this week; I've been so busy and I know my score will not have gone up this time.'

We all want to achieve things in life and putting in hard work with pelvic floor rehabilitation is so much better if you see positive progress. It doesn't matter if pelvic floor rehabilitation takes a while; what is so important is that your motivation remains high. You will get there in the end.

Vaginal Pessaries

Vaginal pessaries should be viewed much like a sports bra; you wouldn't dream of going running without your breasts supported so why not give your vagina the same treatment?

A vaginal pessary is a removable device that is inserted into your vagina, usually by a doctor or women's health specialist. This is to find the correct size and shape of pessary that will work best for you. After the initial fitting you can usually be taught how to put it in and take it out yourself. Most pessaries are made of soft plastic or silicone and come in a variety of shapes and sizes to fit all vaginas. The idea is that it supports the areas that have been affected by the different types of pelvic organ prolapse (see page 54). If you have a prolapse it can be useful to wear a pessary while you are working on your pelvic floor rehabilitation. They give you the freedom to go and walk Hadrian's Wall, if the inclination takes you, without fear of damaging yourself further. Pessaries are a very safe nonsurgical option to treating vaginal prolapse.

They are helpful if you have not finished having children and your prolapse is large and possibly needs a surgical solution (it's usually advised not to have a prolapse repair until you are sure that you have finished your family) and can also be used during pregnancy. They can be particularly helpful in the later stages of pregnancy when your unborn baby is getting heavier and your hormones are making everything more relaxed. So if you feel like everything is falling out please seek help and have a pessary fitted.

Pessaries can be used for the rest of your life, if you wish, and I do have some patients who are doing this and are very happy. It's all about freedom of choice. Whatever you do, don't think that vaginal pessaries are just for the over sixties.

There are very few reasons why pessaries can't be used, such as if you have a pelvic infection or an allergy to the material that pessaries are made from.

A patient of mine with two young children and a very busy job had worked really hard on her pelvic floor rehabilitation. However, the traumatic forceps delivery of her first daughter had stretched her pelvic floor muscles too much. Although her pelvic floor strength was better it was not good enough for her to live her life the way she wanted to live it. So, we discussed the use of a vaginal pessary. She was very happy to give this a go and it has literally given her back her freedom. She is now able to run or stand cooking for hours, which is her passion. After the initial sizing and fitting she was taught how to put it in and take it out (very little difference to a tampon or contraceptive diaphragm), to clean and to change it.

Although this particular woman may require surgery at a later date, at the moment she is very content with life as it is and it gives her a breathing space to plan for the future.

Double Voiding
The idea behind double voiding is to try to empty your bladder more efficiently and it is a useful technique for both men and women. The way to do it is to sit slightly forward on the toilet with your hands on your knees or thighs. Pass urine as best you can, then wait on the toilet for 30 seconds. Lean a bit further

forward (it may help to rock from side to side a bit) then try to pass a bit more urine. Straining to try and force your urine out is not a good idea and if you have a prolapse (see Chapter 5) pushing down to pee may make it worse. Double voiding is a very useful technique to help improve bladder emptying.

Yoga and Pilates

There are many different types of yoga. Yoga originated in ancient India and is now practised all over the world by millions of people.

Pilates is a fitness system developed by a man called Joseph Pilates in the late 1920s in New York to improve balance and strength. Pilates now also has a huge following. Wouldn't it be lovely if 'pelvic floor rehabilitation' had the same ring to it as yoga or Pilates: 'Oh I am just off to do my pelvic floor exercises.'

There is some evidence to suggest that yoga[4] and Pilates[5] can help urinary incontinence, for men as well as women. But at the moment the evidence is to keep doing your pelvic floor rehabilitation as well. Don't rely on yoga and Pilates to cure you by themselves.

Pelvic Floor Exercises for Men

The first thing that you need to do is to become aware of your pelvic floor muscles. You can do this in two stages.

Firstly, the next time you go to have a pee, try to stop the flow of your urine midstream: contract your muscles upward and inward, squeeze, lift and hold. Then let go. Don't worry if the flow did not stop altogether. When you have done this try to keep in your memory which muscles you used to stop the flow. I say this because I don't want you to keep stopping and starting your flow of urine. You should just use this as a test. It can also help to stand naked in front of a mirror – watch the base of your penis; it should appear to be being sucked into your body and your testicles should be moving as though they are contracting up towards your perineum.

The second thing that you need to do is to imagine you are trying to control a bad attack of diarrhoea or imagine you are in a lift full of people and you want to pass wind. Try to pull up the muscles around the back passage or anus.

These muscles that you have been tightening are your pelvic floor muscles. They form the cradle of muscles or hammock that supports your back passage and your urethra. When you perform your pelvic floor exercises you should use all of these muscles at the same time.

HOW TO PERFORM YOUR PELVIC FLOOR EXERCISES

Contract your muscles, squeeze, lift and hold for a count of five (if you can only contract for two seconds then start there) and then gently let go. Now pause for a count of five. Repeat this until you have done five sets of contractions. You should aim to keep your stomach, thigh and buttock muscles relaxed and try to only use your pelvic floor muscles.

It is very important that you do the exercises regularly throughout the day – aim for at least three times a day. It can be helpful to associate doing the exercises with some other activity, so that they become a habit. For example, before you get out of bed in the morning and when you get into bed again at night. Hey presto, you have already done it twice! During the day you could maybe do it when you are driving to work, watching the news or eating your lunch. Without doubt if you have certain daily triggers you will remember to do the exercises much more often.

If you know that you are completely hopeless at remembering to do the exercises, even with prompts, why not download the Squeezy app for men? You can set it to beep at you during the day so there is no excuse whatsoever for forgetting.

Once a day you should also perform a set of ten short, sharp contractions of your pelvic floor. This is done in a rhythmic pattern of squeeze, let go, squeeze, let go.

It is likely to take several weeks before you start to see an improvement. Whatever you do don't give up. Please persevere and continue the exercises even after you start to notice an improvement.

You may find it more difficult to do the exercises in the evening, as your muscles tend to become tired, much like the rest of your body. It's also possible that you notice a mild aching sensation shortly after starting the exercise programme; this is usually due to your muscles getting tired, as with any new fitness regime. The aching in your pelvic floor muscles should subside as your muscles get stronger but if the aching persists just stop doing the exercises for a couple of days.

Electrical Stimulation and PFXA

You can use electrical stimulation to help improve your pelvic floor muscles. There is also something called a PFXA machine; this gives you good biofeedback as it comes with an anal sensor. You put the sensor into your anus, following the instructions, and when you contract your pelvic floor muscles you see a small dial moving from 1 to 12. As always it's motivating to see progress. Women can also use this device (with either a vaginal or anal sensor) if they wish.

PART TWO

Tackling Problems

THREE

Will I Ever Trampoline Again?
How to Understand and Tackle
Stress Incontinence

The muscles of the pelvic floor support the bladder and keep us dry. Stress incontinence happens when these muscles become weak and the neck of your bladder does not always stay closed under stress, which then leads to urine leaks. Stress incontinence commonly occurs after childbirth or the menopause but it can also occur if you have had gynaecological surgery, for example a hysterectomy. In men, it's more common after procedures to correct issues with the prostate, especially prostate cancer.

Research indicates that between 25 and 45 per cent of women around the world suffer from stress incontinence[6] although, it should be noted, these are just the women who are willing to admit it. The large statistical variance is almost certainly due to many people being too embarrassed to be completely honest about their symptoms. Imagine if you were asked if you had any symptoms of incontinence after having your baby and perhaps occasionally you do (maybe just when you sneeze) – what would you say? I hope that after reading this you will feel empowered to proudly say, yes, I have and I am doing something about it.

What is Stress Incontinence?

Stress incontinence is an entirely physical issue that is not in any way related to mental stress or anxiety. It usually happens when you cough, sneeze, laugh or run. Sometimes it can be very minor indeed and only happens when you put your pelvic floor under extra stress, for example, when trampolining or skipping. Many of my patients over the years had spent a very long time assuming that these sorts of leaks were entirely normal before they finally came to see me. It is not and should never be thought of as normal! If you suffer from even minor stress incontinence it is really important to address it sooner rather than later – do not leave it until that awkward moment when your ten-year-old asks you to skip down the street with them or join them on the trampoline.

I often think of one of my lovely patients who decided to follow a rather strenuous exercise video one afternoon to get back into shape after overindulging at Christmas. She gave it her best shot but sure enough, disaster struck – she had awful stress incontinence (mercifully on a wooden floor). At that very moment the doorbell rang. She quickly pulled on a large jumper and opened the door to the local vicar. As you can imagine she was completely horrified and stunned but she let the vicar in. Both of them looked at the puddle before she quickly ushered the vicar into the sitting room saying, 'Bad dog! How could you have weed in the house?' Mercifully he didn't stay very long and the dog was given a treat! When she recounted this story we both laughed – it could almost be a comedy sketch. You'll be pleased to know that she has since given up the exercise video for more pelvic floor-friendly exercises in the form of long walks with her dog, while also working hard on rehabilitating her pelvic floor. I hope it doesn't take something as drastic as this to get you motivated into action!

Sometimes stress incontinence can be so bad that simply standing up from a sitting position can cause a leak of urine or it may only happen with a very bad cough or a massive sneeze. I am sure you have all heard people say, 'I laughed so much I wet myself,' but if you've ever experienced any of this in real life, it's stress incontinence and needs attention. It's shocking how many women see mild incontinence as normal and are putting up with the problem. So many women tell me, 'Oh, I always have spare knickers with me, you know, just in case.'

I hope that if your symptoms are worse than that then you will have already sought some help. But if your symptoms are milder please don't be complacent – it is vital that you start pelvic floor rehabilitation now.

How Do I Tell if I Have Stress Incontinence?

- Have you ever had to stop in the street to cross your legs before you sneeze?
- Have you stopped running, playing tennis or any other sport that you really enjoyed because you're worried you might have an accident?

If so, then you are suffering from stress incontinence. It is very sad that stress incontinence, or any type of incontinence for that matter, is still such a taboo subject. It is embarrassing but it is nothing to be ashamed about – the most important thing is that you seek help so let's end this taboo now.

I regularly see women who tell me, 'No, I don't have any incontinence,' but when I ask them whether they lack the confidence to sneeze, run, jump or – horror of horrors – trampoline, the response is usually, 'Yes, that's definitely me.' Once the realization hits, their next words are almost always, 'What on earth is wrong with me, why am I in denial? I should have dealt with this years ago.'

While incontinence remains such a taboo it's hardly surprising that so many of us are firmly in denial. If this subject ever comes up it's generally after a few glasses of wine or a night out with close girlfriends and a good giggle, mostly with everyone saying, 'I must sort this out, really I must.'

Breaking the Taboo

I'm pleased to say that pelvic floor issues are a regular discussion point at almost every dinner party I attend. Inevitably I will be sitting next to a man, who after a while will say, 'What do you do?' When I tell him it's usually not at all what he was expecting! This is generally after a few glasses of wine and a good meal and, almost inevitably, the whole table starts to talk about what I do – on more than one occasion the evening has been spent in in-depth discussion about vaginas and the pelvic floor.

The quotes below are from just a small selection of my patients over the years:

I am sure I will be OK – this is just a temporary problem, isn't it?

When I stop breastfeeding and my hormones return to normal it will be OK, won't it?

I don't want to end up like my mum, wearing pads all the time.

How can my body be so fit yet I leak when I run?

I have been doing Pilates for years – my pelvic floor must be super-strong, surely?

There is a lot of research that looks at female athletes and stress incontinence. One particular study found that between 28 and 80 per cent of female athletes suffered from urinary incontinence.[7] The high figures of 80 per cent were found in women who do things like gymnastics and trampolining. So if you are a young, fit and healthy woman who hasn't had any children but is regularly doing high-impact sports activities such as running, netball, aerobics and HIIT, please don't assume that stress incontinence is a problem of the over-fifties; whatever your age and level of fitness this is the moment to start the revolution. With so many more of us now involved in high-impact sports, it's even more important to make pelvic floor exercises part of your routine now to avoid significant problems later in life.

I recently had a patient who had just had a baby. She wanted to get her body back into shape following the birth so she booked some sessions with a personal trainer in order to get 'bikini fit' for an upcoming holiday. Unfortunately in the first session he made her perform star jumps on a mini trampoline and, of course, she had terrible stress incontinence. Mercifully black Lycra can hide most catastrophes!

It's so important to include your pelvic floor as part of your overall health and fitness; it's just as important to get that back into shape after pregnancy if you want to stay active throughout your life.

Solving Stress Incontinence

The most important thing we need to do to prevent and tackle stress incontinence is to incorporate pelvic floor exercises into our daily routine. They can be done anywhere and at any time but the challenge is remembering to do them regularly and, more importantly, properly. This is what I hear every day:

How do I know if I am doing the exercises properly?

Please refer back to Chapter 2 to check how to find, isolate and exercise your pelvic floor muscles. If you simply can't find them please go and see a professional to help get you started.

We've all heard about pelvic floor exercises and I am sure that most women who have had a baby or any kind of gynaecological surgery were given a leaflet about them. How many of you have that leaflet filed away nice and safe? Maybe it's in your 'to do' pile? Do you still have it at all? If it's something you've put to the back of your mind I do have every sympathy for you. When you have a new baby to take care of, and especially as a first-time mother, your whole world has changed so unless you have very bad stress incontinence or a prolapse, pelvic floor exercises are in all likelihood a low priority.

Pelvic floor exercises are something that everyone should be doing but I know the reality is that we are not doing them as often as we should (if at all) on a daily basis. Maybe you remember to do them if you have a bad cough or it's hay fever season (and by the way, bladder problems are more common than hay fever) but I suspect that many of you might have started to do a few but then given up. And more importantly, are you doing the exercises correctly?

There are many variations of pelvic floor exercises and if you look online you'll find pages and pages of websites telling you lots of different, often very confusing things. So the first thing to remember is to keep it simple and consider the simple advice I have outlined in Chapter 2. The primary focus should be on building a habit that you can incorporate into your daily routine without totally disrupting your life, or worse, making you feel that you have failed to stick to the plan, to the extent that you become despondent and give up. That would be truly tragic.

Numerous studies show that if you have help or supervision while doing your pelvic floor exercises then greater improvement occurs.[8] Following some of the instructions in Chapter 2 should lead you in the right direction for recovery of your muscle tone. But if you are still struggling after that then please seek the help of a women's health physiotherapist or a specialist continence nurse.

There are also surgical solutions for stress incontinence but please don't consider this route until you have tried conservative treatments first. You might surprise yourself with how well you do and in the short term you have nothing to lose. If you do end up being referred by your doctor to a specialist for surgery then keep doing your pelvic floor exercises. Even if they haven't cured you they will still help you to continue to build up muscle strength while you wait – and you may well find that the problem is solved before you end up in the operating theatre.

Things to Watch Out for During Rehabilitation

While you are in the process of strengthening your pelvic floor, you should try to avoid doing things that will slow down your recovery, or that could even make your problems worse. These are:

- Running or jogging, particularly on hard pavements. If it's something you absolutely can't give up then switch to running on grass or a treadmill, which may lessen the impact on your pelvic floor. You could try wearing either a large tampon or a menstrual cup, such as a Mooncup or Ruby Cup. There are also vaginal pessaries available to buy online – Contam, Contrelle Activgard and Contiform, to name but three. These usually come in a starter pack of three different sizes; you can try them out to see which one works best for you before buying a pack of the correct size. All these things work by applying gentle pressure to the neck of your bladder and, hey presto, you should be able to run without leaking.
- Lifting heavy weights – and this does include large toddlers!
- Straining on the toilet with constipation (I'll tackle some aspects of this in Chapter 9).
- Being overweight. Carrying excess weight, particularly around the abdomen, puts pressure on your pelvic floor so this could well be the moment to do something about those extra pounds you've put on.
- Lots of coughing, so if you smoke this may be a good time to quit (see Helpful Organizations, page 155).

Giggle Incontinence

Urinary incontinence can affect young and teenage girls too and is commonly called 'giggle incontinence'. It is not a terribly well understood phenomenon but is thought to be caused by an overactive bladder. If it is very severe it can be treated with drugs to calm your bladder. As always, the first thing to do is to learn to do pelvic floor exercises as this may help you to brace and contract your muscles if you are about to giggle and may help to stop the leakage. If you (as it can persist into adulthood) or your daughter is suffering from this issue you can find more information in the Helpful Organizations section on page 156, including details of a YouTube video about pelvic floor rehabilitation for teenagers.

Encouraging young people to talk about, embrace and understand their bodies is slowly happening. When I was at school my girlfriends and I didn't chat to each other about periods. I spent half the time checking the back of my skirt, terrified I might have started without realizing. These days young girls are much more aware – many of them even plot their periods on an app, which they can discuss with their friends. They are more open and learn every day from things that they read and see on the internet. I believe that if young people understood the importance of their pelvic floor muscles and pelvic floor health early on, this would be a great step forward for their future wellbeing, and I think young women would start to be more open about it. As it happens, I know that this is starting to happen, among young twenty-somethings. A little bird told me that the editorial office in charge of publishing my book (which is largely made up of young women) are now openly talking about pelvic floor and bladder issues, things that would have never been mentioned before. This fills my heart with joy – it's the start of the revolution!

I don't treat children but whenever young women come to see me they love the Squeezy app (see page 17); they always embrace it as it makes the exercises so much easier – and gives helpful reminders. I've learned that printed leaflets with pelvic floor exercises are probably not going to cut it with younger women, while older women probably still appreciate them. What I am trying to say here is that it's important to pick a treatment or an approach that fits with your lifestyle.

Mixed Urinary Incontinence

This happens when you have both stress incontinence and urinary urge incontinence (see Chapter 4 for more on this condition). If you have symptoms of both but you are otherwise well with, for example, no urinary infections, then the first line of treatment is pelvic floor rehabilitation. I regularly have patients who come to see me with stress incontinence; even when I ask them if they have any urinary urgency they report that they don't. What I find very interesting is that often when they come back for review, I often hear, 'My stress incontinence is getting better, but amazingly I am not hopping up and down on my doorstep any more desperate for the toilet.' So often they don't realize that they had a problem until it has gone away.

FOUR

Rushing to the Loo: the Overactive Bladder and Urge Incontinence

The Overactive Bladder

Do you either frequently or constantly need to pass urine, even if you went only half an hour ago? Are you someone who knows where every toilet in your hometown is? Do you dread the thought of long car journeys? Are you the one whose children say, 'Oh, Mum, you don't need the loo again, do you?'

Perhaps you have found yourself crossing your legs on the doorstep, frantically searching in the bottom of your handbag for the door keys and hopping up and down in a bid to get the key in the door so you can get into the house before disaster strikes. A lot of people find that even the sight of their front door makes them desperate for the toilet. Or sometimes the trigger might be just turning into your street and sensing that you are nearly home. Not being able to get to the toilet in time can really affect your quality of life.

Do you have a sudden urgent desire to pass urine often completely out of the blue? One minute you are totally fine and the next you are absolutely desperate to pee. This can then turn into urge incontinence.

What is Urge Incontinence?

Urge incontinence happens when the initial urgent desire to go to the toilet overwhelms you and you simply can't hold on, at which point you leak. The leakage can be minimal, in the form of a very small wet patch in your underwear, or it can be your bladder completely emptying. If it is the latter then it doesn't matter where you are, it is horrifying. A feeling of total lack of control of a bodily function of any kind is shocking but there is no hiding from this. If any of the situations mentioned above are familiar to you then you could be suffering from an overactive bladder.

If you suffer from urge incontinence then it may well be that you have stopped going out, turning down invitations from your friends as a result of these problems. How often have you given the excuse: 'Oh I'm a bit busy today, I'll come next time'? Or perhaps, when you do go out you only go to places where you know you'll have easy access to a toilet. Do you always sit at the end of the row in the cinema because being trapped in the middle of the row fills you with dread?

Are you getting up at night to go to the toilet more than once? This can be exhausting and having disturbed sleep patterns makes the next day that much harder. If you share a bed your frequent trips to the bathroom are probably disturbing your partner, resulting in everyone feeling cross and upset. This can happen as a result of going to the toilet too frequently during the day so that your bladder capacity shrinks. Or in men it could be caused by an enlarged prostate gland. Whatever the cause, you don't have to put up with it and there are lots of ways of sorting it out.

Why Does Overactive Bladder and Urge Incontinence Happen?

In some cases there is no reason why your bladder starts to misbehave and the cause may be unknown. This is often true for young people; believe me, it affects both young men and women, far more than you think. If you are young it's an especially terrible and baffling problem. Who on earth do you go to for help and where do you start seeking advice? Can you even discuss this with your family or closest friends? I'm sure some of you have had a sneaky peek on the internet and either terrified yourself, or just got confused as to what is wrong and what to do about it.

The root cause can sometimes just be a case of habit. Maybe it started during an anxious period in your life and the toilet became almost a sanctuary or place to hide: 'Just popping to the loo' becomes a way to get out of or away from difficult situations. Suddenly it's a problem not a habit. Going to the toilet 'just in case' is a little secret for millions of people. I often tell my patients that their bladder is controlling their lives; the solution is to put you back in control.

Then there is the fear that you might wet yourself. This can create a pattern of going to the toilet frequently to make sure that it doesn't happen. It can become progressively worse as you get into the habit of rushing off to the toilet when you feel the slightest sensation of wanting to pass urine. This can sometimes happen when you have an existing problem. I have had lots of male patients who have had stress incontinence following a radical prostatectomy and in their bid to pre-empt leaks they have started going too frequently. As a result when their stress incontinence is better they end up with a different problem of urinary frequency and decreased bladder capacity. They then have to do some bladder training to restore normal functioning.

Sometimes it is simply the result of the ageing process, with mobility making it more difficult to get to the toilet in time. It can also be caused by recurrent urine infections (or even a one-off infection), which leave you exhausted and unwell and, on top of it all, running to the toilet every five minutes. Sometimes the cause can be certain medications that you are taking or an illness like multiple sclerosis or Parkinson's disease. Urge incontinence can sometimes happen after a stroke.

Vaginal prolapse in the form of cystocele (front wall vaginal prolapse) is another culprit. If you think this is you, keep reading, but do also look at Chapter 5 on pelvic organ prolapse, as you will need to refer to both to fully understand the issues at hand. In men it can also happen when you have an enlarged prostate and your bladder isn't emptying very well – please take a look at Chapter 10 for more information.

When you suffer from urge incontinence or overactive bladder then it can be distressing; you don't look ill, and in most cases you are not ill. However, it's hard to be the one constantly getting up and rushing off to the loo. I looked after a judge some time ago with this problem and as you can imagine stopping court proceedings every half an hour is not on at all. When he was better he told me, 'I will never stop people leaving my court again to go to the toilet.' In general we are very intolerant of people's toilet habits and I think that's due to our own fears and lack of understanding of the problem. We're going to run through some solutions here but while you are on the road to recovery you can obtain a card called the 'Just Can't Wait' card which provides clear and discreet communication that you need to use the toilet urgently (see Helpful Organizations, page 160). This may not be for everyone but it could get you out of a difficult situation if needed.

What is Normal?
On average we should go to the toilet to pass urine between 6 and 8 times per day, passing about 300ml each time, though at times it could be as much as 400–600ml. This may also include once at night.

We all vary as human beings, and our understanding of normal can be greatly affected by outside influences. I once treated a patient in her twenties who was at the end of her tether as she was getting a lot of hostile looks and comments in the office, such as 'Off to the loo again, what's wrong with you?' It was seen as a sign of laziness or trying to get out of work. Amazingly, no one batted an eyelid when the smokers said with a giggle, 'Just nipping out for a breath of fresh air!' The poor woman had started to think up excuses like going to get a drink of water (via the loo) or doing some photocopying (via the loo). It was such a problem but she had not considered how to fix it until she came to see me. During our consultation she confided in me that she was drinking about eight cans of caffeinated fizzy drink a day. After giving these up and doing some bladder training and pelvic floor exercise she was completely back to normal. However, she had suffered totally unnecessarily for over a year without seeking help.

There is definitely a link between consuming caffeinated drinks and increased urinary frequency. However, there is no need to miss your morning cup of tea – I would never be so cruel as to suggest that! One or two cups of tea or coffee a day will not make a huge difference but if you know that your double espresso makes you have horrible urgency then you will have to think about cutting down on your coffee consumption.

I remember one patient of mine who had recently retired. He was now at home all day spending a lot of time in the garden. His wife was a big tea drinker and she was now making a cup for him every time she had one. He wasn't used to all this tea but he didn't really think anything of it until he started to go to the toilet a lot and have some urinary urgency. He came to seek my help for his new and distressing problem. Having made the connection with his huge increase in tea drinking we decided this was the likely culprit, but if stopping the tea wasn't the answer then further tests could be pursued. He just hadn't connected drinking tea with his new bladder problems. Needless to say he is now cured.

Alcohol can also be a factor and we are increasingly aware of the need to drink alcohol in moderation, for all sorts of health reasons (if you are unsure whether your intake is within safe levels then you can find further information and some useful calculators at drinkaware.co.uk). However, you might not have considered the effects on your bladder function. Admitting to drinking a bit too much alcohol is often one of the things that people confide in me and urge incontinence can be the trigger not only to reducing your drinking but also being generally healthier, with the benefit of improved bladder function an added bonus.

Another thing that I hear and read all the time is that we should all drink plenty of water. It has become the norm to walk about clutching a large bottle of water – we are even told in train and tube stations to carry water with us in hot weather. This is fine as we don't want people fainting on the train – but how much is plenty?

We should drink 1.5–2 litres of fluid per day. If you are doing large amounts of exercise, then adding in an extra 500ml of fluid is a good idea. Remember that you will usually pass more urine than the fluid that you have drunk, as there is also water in the food you eat. So don't be alarmed if you pass out more urine than fluid that you drank – though of course you will only be aware of this if you start measuring the amounts. A good rule of thumb is to check the colour of your urine – it should be a pale straw colour. Let's say it should look more like champagne than beer!

Drinking too little can also be a problem. I see many patients who tell me that they don't drink all day if they are going out, in case they can't get to a loo. This is just as bad as drinking too much, as drinking too little can lead to strong concentrated urine that irritates an ever-shrinking bladder, meaning that even those who are drinking very little are going to the loo every half an hour as their bladders have shrunk.

However, all is not lost and there are easy solutions to this very curable problem. Once you realize that your bladder has taken on a demanding and distressing life of its own, totally ruling you and your life, you can start to take back control and show your bladder who's boss.

BLADDER RETRAINING

The first and simplest solution for an overactive bladder is bladder retraining. The great thing about bladder retraining is that there are no side effects so it's a great place to start. Most of you will be able to do this on your own following the simple rules below but as always if you are struggling please seek the help of a specialist nurse or physiotherapist.

The aim of bladder retraining is to steadily lengthen the time between your visits to the toilet, while ensuring that your fluid intake is not reduced in any way.

The first step is to keep a bladder diary (you can use the one on the Squeezy app if you like). Write down how often you have passed urine over a few days, remembering to note down any middle-of-the-night trips to the toilet, as well as how many drinks you have had. If you wish you can get a more accurate idea of what is going on by measuring your fluid intake and urine output. Measuring intake isn't too much of a problem, once you work out how much your mugs and glasses hold, but it's probably best to do this on a day when you are at home with plenty of privacy if you're going to accurately measure your urine output. Find an old measuring jug (or buy one specifically for this purpose – the cook of the household might not look kindly on you using their best measuring jug!) to pee into and then make a note of the volume of liquid. A bladder diary can be quite an eye-opener; for example, if you are going to the toilet fifteen times a day and each time only passing 100ml, you can then see immediately that something is very definitely wrong. Even if you knew that you were going far too often, writing it down makes it much more real.

The diary is the starting point to training your bladder to return to its normal functioning. It is useful to keep the diary for about three days at the beginning of the bladder training and then repeat this after a couple of weeks. You can then compare the two diaries to see if you are making progress. Some people like to keep a diary all the time through the training so just do whatever works for you.

The next step is to try to increase the length of time between your visits to the toilet. When you get the urge to pass urine, try to hold on for a short period of time before going to the toilet, starting with five minutes. Sometimes sitting on a hard seat may help; it might take your mind off the urge to pee by applying pressure to your perineum. You can sit down and try to do a few pelvic floor contractions. This might reduce or take away the urge to pass urine for a while. Even trying to think of other things can help.

When you have managed this for a few days then you can try to gradually increase the time you hold on for from 5 minutes to 10 minutes, and so on from there. The increase in the time you hold on should be slow and gradual. Do not try to rush things by holding on for too long; if you force it you may end up with an incontinence episode, which would be a shame and may put you off the whole process. Slow and steady is the way forward.

The whole process is likely to take between one and three months to complete. After this you should find that you need to pass urine about every 3–4 hours during the day, and perhaps once at night, passing 250–300ml each time, or possibly a bit more. You will know it has worked if you are now living your life without worrying about where the nearest toilet is.

A lot of people find the nights a problem but rest assured that if you take care of the day the night should take care of itself. Your bladder will have expanded so you will be able to sleep for longer before your bladder sends that message to your brain that it is full.

Alongside bladder retraining it is important that you continue to practise your pelvic floor exercises (see Chapter 2), as these are crucial to helping your recovery. And now might be the time to take a look at your diet. Eating plenty of fruit, vegetables and other foods containing fibre is key as constipation can make an already overactive bladder worse.

Other foods that may affect your bladder include chocolate, acidic fruit and vegetables like oranges, grapefruits, lemons and tomatoes, artificial sweeteners, spicy food and raw onion. As previously mentioned, tea, coffee, alcohol, and fizzy and carbonated drinks (including fizzy water) can all irritate your bladder. It may be a good idea to keep a food diary if you are unsure which foods are upsetting your bladder, or it may be that you already know in your heart that the curry you occasionally treat yourself to makes your symptoms worse. Try to work out what food or drink is affecting you and then do your best to eliminate it from your diet.

What if It Doesn't Work?

If you have tried the above and are still struggling then the next step is to consider medication to reboot your bladder to behave itself. It's not that you haven't worked hard enough at your exercises but more likely that your bladder is having unexplained spasms that you cannot control. Bladder spasms can be treated with specific drugs that work on the smooth muscle of your bladder to calm it down, enabling you to 'hold on' for longer.

You will need to make an appointment to see your GP if you think that medication is the way forward for you. Depending on the advice from your doctor you can sometimes use the medication in conjunction with bladder retraining and pelvic floor exercises so that after two or three months you may well be able to discontinue the drug. Equally, you may need to take the medication on an ongoing basis. If this is the case you need to see it like any other medication; if it is giving you back your lost quality of life, it is the best way forward.

I saw a woman a while ago who had collected for the Lifeboats charity (RNLI) every year for the last twenty years. She came to see me heartbroken that she wouldn't be able to continue with this as the area she had to collect in had no toilets nearby. She was trying pelvic floor exercises and bladder retraining but was still struggling, so I recommended that she try medication as well and this worked a treat. We are all different and if one thing doesn't work for you another thing will, so whatever you do don't give up until you find the answer.

Other Solutions

If the bladder retraining isn't making enough of a difference and you don't want to take pills then you could try tibial nerve stimulation. This is a minimally invasive clinic-based procedure that has been shown to be safe and effective in treating overactive bladder symptoms.[9] The treatment involves having a fine acupuncture needle inserted in your ankle, which is then connected to a small stimulation unit that stimulates the tibial nerve with gentle electrical impulses. The mild current is then carried to the nerves that control bladder function and hopefully calms the overactive bladder. You need to attend the clinic once a week for twelve consecutive weeks and each treatment takes 30 minutes, so this option does require a lot of commitment.

There is also something called sacral nerve stimulation or sacral neuromodulation therapy. This involves implanting a small stimulation device under the skin, usually at the top of your buttock or in the lower abdomen. The machine delivers electrical stimulation to the sacral nerve and this stimulation can help to stop unwanted messages from the bladder that you are desperate to pass urine. The device will last for five to ten years before it needs replacing. It's worth noting that new treatments are being developed all the time to help with overactive bladder so you need to keep a lookout or ask your GP to refer you to a urologist.

There are also some more radical medical treatments for the overactive bladder. However, these treatments should really only be considered when all else has failed.

Botox is commonly used as a cosmetic treatment; injected into the face to help reduce wrinkles. In the same way Botox can be used to relax the muscles of the bladder and help to calm it down. The procedure is carried out in a hospital and is performed with either a local or general anaesthetic. It is a relatively quick procedure usually done as a day case or with an overnight stay in hospital. You may have to have repeat injections and this could be at intervals anywhere between six and eighteen months after the procedure if your symptoms recur.

Another option – and this really is a last resort – is to undergo surgery to increase the size of your bladder. The procedure is performed under a general anaesthetic and can be performed laparoscopically or as an open operation. This is usually done by cutting open your bladder and sewing a piece of your intestine into the opening, increasing your bladder capacity. In general it will take at least six weeks to recover from this type of surgery.

Dealing with Incontinence

So far in this chapter we have focused on urinary frequency and urgency but not on actual incontinence. This is where the world of the incontinence pad comes into play.

I have no doubt that you have all seen the huge variety that is now on sale in pharmacies, supermarkets and on the internet. They come as disposable or reusable and in all shapes and sizes. These are specially designed to do the job, yet lots of women are still buying sanitary towels instead. I often see women who are without doubt past the menopause and are definitely not still having any periods with sanitary pads in their supermarket trolley. This again suggests at least a denial of the problem and at worst conforming to the taboo and shame that people associate with incontinence. It really has to stop.

While you are taking other steps to improving your incontinence, pads certainly help to deal with the problem, but it is important to see pads as a temporary aid, only to be used while you are curing the problem. Sometimes pads are advertised or presented as a solution to the problem. THEY ARE NOT. I often come across people wearing two pads one on top of the other; this is hopeless as the pads have a plastic backing and urine can't flow between the two, so you need to find one single pad that does the job for you.

Urinary Tract Infections

Although urinary tract infections are not directly related to an overactive bladder the two things often have the symptoms of urinary frequency and urgency in common. It's important that you find out what your problem is so you can successfully sort it out. Urinary tract infections (often known as UTIs or cystitis) plague some women's lives while others have never had one. They are the second most common type of infection after chest infections. The most common cause of UTI is bacteria from your anus getting into your urethra, although this has nothing to do with poor hygiene – it's much more common in women due to our much shorter urethra and its proximity to our bottom.

If you have a urine infection then you may have suddenly started having some incontinence; you will usually experience urgency and frequency in going to the toilet. UTIs can be painful; you may have the shivers and feel really pretty rotten. You may also have blood in your urine or cloudy urine. A urine test is a good idea to find out exactly which type of bacteria is causing the problem and also to help rule out that something else isn't causing your symptoms. The vital thing is to be treated with the correct antibiotic. This is very important, particularly in a world where bacteria are becoming increasingly resistant to antibiotics.

You can try a variety of over-the-counter treatments like D-mannose, probiotics, ascorbic acid (vitamin C), potassium citrate and cranberry juice. There is some positive evidence to suggest that these remedies can help you but it's important to note that none of it is hugely conclusive. I would always suggest that you seek advice from your doctor or pharmacist before taking any home remedies as these may react adversely with any other medication that you might also be taking.

How to help prevent cystitis and other UTIs:

- Always have a wee after sex.
- Make sure your fluid intake is 1.5–2 litres per day.
- Wipe your bottom from front to back.
- Don't have baths all the time or use scented products in the bath water.
- Wear cotton underwear.
- Avoid skintight jeans.
- Have a look at your birth control; it might be that the spermicidal lubrication is to blame.

Interstitial Cystitis or Bladder Pain Syndrome

This is a chronic condition where inflammation of your bladder causes pain. At the moment no one really knows what causes it. It can cause awful pelvic pain and strong feelings of urinary urgency or frequency both during the day and at night. It might be worse during menstruation and after sexual intercourse. It tends to happen more to middle-aged women but as with all things it can happen to anyone.

It is quite difficult to diagnose and also difficult to treat. Often you would need a cystoscopy (a camera to look inside your bladder). If you have a diagnosis of interstitial cystitis you can receive very helpful advice from an organization called Bladder Health UK (see Helpful Organizations, page 159).

It's important to note that you may suffer from overactive bladder and stress incontinence at the same time. This is called mixed urinary incontinence and to treat it you will need to do pelvic floor rehabilitation as well as following the advice in this chapter, so please refer back to Chapters 2 and 3 for more information.

FIVE

Everything Feels Like It Might Fall Out: Types of Vaginal Prolapse

Pelvic organ prolapse (POP) or vaginal prolapse has been described in medical texts since the very beginning of time. What they did to women to help with prolapse would make our hair stand on end now!

Hippocrates (*c.* 460–377 BC) thought that the best way to treat prolapse would be to place pleasant fumes near a woman's head and vile ones near her prolapsed womb in order to stimulate the uterus to retreat. If that didn't work then half a pomegranate soaked in vinegar was placed in the vagina to keep the prolapse in place. And if that didn't work then the poor woman was dangled upside down with her feet attached to a wooden frame that was then bounced repeatedly. She was then put on a bed with her legs tied together for three days.[10&11] The upside-down treatment was actually quite sensible as in the short term it would have caused the prolapse to retreat back into the vagina. However, the results would always have been short-lived once the woman started moving around normally as gravity would cause the prolapse to descend once more.

By the end of the sixteenth century there was extensive use of vaginal pessaries made of a variety of materials such as brass, cork, wood, wax, leather, glass or metal. Although these might have held the prolapse in place they must have caused awful infections and been very uncomfortable to wear.

In the mid- to late-nineteenth century chloroform started to be used as a general anaesthetic (Queen Victoria had it administered for the birth of two of her children, Prince Leopold in 1853 and Princess Beatrice in 1857, which had the effect of leading people to accept the safety of anaesthesia) and surgery started to happen more frequently. However, it was not until the improvements in asepsis that more advanced surgery could be performed. By the 1950s surgery started to become a real option for women with prolapse, giving them the choice of how to be best treated.

With good pelvic floor rehabilitation and the use of modern pessaries women now have plenty of options before going down the surgical route. However, the surgical advances that have been made in areas such as laparoscopic and vaginal surgery mean that a surgical solution for your prolapse may be offered, if needed.

It is entirely possible with pelvic floor rehabilitation to get your prolapse to a point where, although it may be still there, it's not bothering you and doesn't interfere with your daily life. If this is the case you can then decide to continue like this and avoid surgery for the moment, knowing that it is an option if you need it later on.

What is a Prolapse?

A prolapse happens when the muscles and ligaments of your pelvic floor are weakened. The condition occurs when, because of weakened pelvic floor muscles and a weakened vaginal wall, one or more of the pelvic organs, most commonly the bladder, bulges into the vagina. Before I explore the causes I will explain the various types of prolapse that occur along with levels of severity. Then we will look at what can cause prolapse and how to treat it.

Having a prolapse can be distressing and can really affect your quality of life but don't despair – please read on so you can hopefully start on the road to recovery.

If you haven't yet been examined by your doctor or women's health specialist, this guide may help you figure out the type and severity of the prolapse you might have. I hope that it will help you to understand what is happening to your body so you can start trying to manage your prolapse before you seek professional help.

It is thought that about 50 per cent of women over fifty have some degree or symptoms of prolapse, although it should be noted that, as with most problems in this area, these are just the women who have reported the problem. A prolapse may have no symptoms and only be noticed on a routine smear test. So please, even if you don't have any symptoms of prolapse, start your pelvic floor muscle training today.

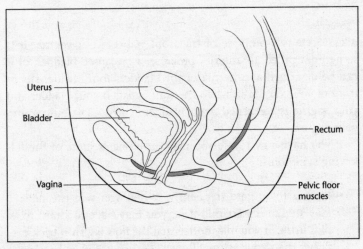

Pelvic organs in the correct position

Before we start looking at what can happen to us when we have a prolapse, here are a few reflections from some of my patients:

It feels like I am sitting on an egg or a ball.

It feels like something is falling out.

I have had three urine infections and I have never suffered with them before.

I have started to have awful constipation recently.

I have stopped running as it feels so uncomfortable.

I don't want to have sex, it is embarrassing with this prolapse there.

Types of Prolapse

Prolapse comes in various forms and I have listed the most commonly occurring ones below:

Cystocele

A cystocele is a prolapse of the front wall of your vagina. It is sometimes called an anterior prolapse, a prolapsed bladder, or it can be described as a hernia of the bladder. Your bladder sits in front of your vagina so when the wall between your bladder and your vagina is weakened, your bladder protrudes or bulges into your vagina.

If you have a cystocele you may have one or more of the following symptoms:

- Having to urinate frequently. When you wee the flow may stop and start mid-flow, you may have to strain to pass urine or you may notice that the flow is a thin trickle rather than your normal flow.

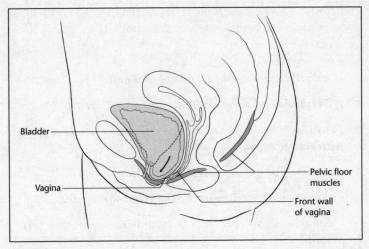

Cystocele

- You may have to sit on the toilet waiting for the urine to start flowing due to your bladder not being in its normal place any more.
- You may also have an urgent need to pass urine and a feeling that you haven't fully emptied your bladder, which means a return visit to the toilet half an hour later.
- You may notice a bulge in your vagina, or sometimes you may have a feeling of heaviness in that area.
- You may start getting more urinary tract infections.
- You may have found that sex has become painful or uncomfortable or are experiencing urinary incontinence during sex.

Rectocele

A rectocele is a prolapse of the back wall of your vagina. It is sometimes called a posterior vaginal wall prolapse, or a hernia of your bowel. It happens when your rectum bulges into your vagina. This happens when the wall between your rectum and your vagina is weakened and can be made worse if you lost part of your

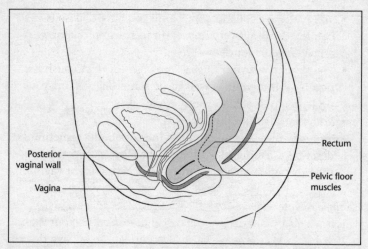

Rectocele

perineum during childbirth (see Chapter 6). When this happens there is not enough support for the back wall of your vagina, making it easier for a rectocele to bulge downwards.

If you have a rectocele you may have one or more of the following symptoms:

- You may find emptying your bowels more difficult and have been straining on the toilet. I see women all the time who have been using all sorts of ways of emptying their bowels from medication to suppositories to colonic irrigation without looking at the prolapse that is the root of the problem. I suspect there are a number of reasons for this: not knowing where to go for help; thinking it's normal or maybe having been told it's normal ('what do you expect, you've had two children'); definitely feeling too shy or embarrassed to talk about it.
- You may have a feeling that you haven't emptied your bowels properly.

- You may have constipation where you have had no issues before. It's always very important to see your doctor with any change in your bowel habits.
- You have to put your fingers into your vagina to push the poo back into your bowels (as it sometimes sits in your prolapse) to be able to empty them.
- You may be finding sex painful.
- You may have a feeling of heaviness (patients sometimes describe a feeling like having a heavily soaked tampon in their vagina) or a pressure in your perineum or vagina.

Uterine Prolapse

This is when your uterus (womb) descends down into your vagina.

If you have a uterine prolapse (descent) you may have the following symptoms:

- You may have a feeling of heaviness in your vagina like a lump coming down.

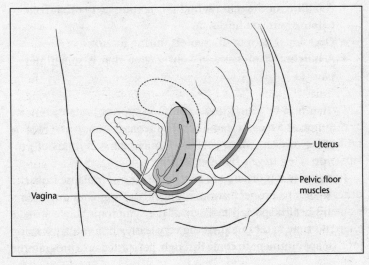

Uterine prolapse

- Having intercourse may cause a painful feeling deep inside your vagina.
- If the descent of your uterus is very severe your cervix may be at the entrance to your vagina or protruding out at this point. The prolapse may be so bad that your cervix is rubbing on your pants. At this point you feel like everything is falling out.
- You may start having some urinary incontinence.

Vaginal Vault Prolapse

This can happen when you have had a hysterectomy and the top of your vagina (where your cervix and uterus were) descends down into your vagina.

Enterocele

An enterocele is when your small bowel pushes into your vagina. It is less common than other types of prolapse. Symptoms include:

- Lower back pain
- A pulling or dragging sensation in your vagina that feels better when you lie down
- Occasional pain or discomfort during intercourse
- A bulging or pressure in your vagina that is sometimes painful

Cystocele is by far the most common type of prolapse – twice as common as a rectocele and three times as common as a uterine prolapse. However, when you have quite bad symptoms of prolapse you often have a bit of each type.

In any case it is often hard to tell one type of prolapse from the other without a proper examination, either from your doctor or a women's health specialist. If any of the symptoms above strike a chord it's time to seek help. At the very least, while you are waiting for that appointment to come through, get started on a programme of pelvic floor rehabilitation; you may find that your symptoms improve quite quickly.

General Symptoms of Prolapse

A prolapse often feels worse after standing for long periods, at the end of a busy day (particularly when you are running around after your children) or lifting anything heavy. Your prolapse is usually least troublesome first thing in the morning after you have been lying down all night sleeping or resting, for obvious reasons of gravity (that's why that ancient 'cure' of dangling women upside down followed by bed rest worked so well in the short term – not that I'm suggesting this as an option!). When you have been in bed all night there has been less downward pressure on your prolapse so it will have retreated back inside – until you start rushing about with your busy day.

Here are some of the symptoms you may be experiencing if you have a prolapse:

- An aching feeling in the lower part of your abdomen
- Difficulty inserting tampons
- Feeling uncomfortable when you cough, strain or bear down
- Urinary incontinence in the form of stress incontinence, urinary frequency or urge incontinence (see chapters 3 and 4)
- Pain, pressure, discomfort or leaking urine during sexual intercourse, leading to you not wanting to have intercourse. If this is happening it may help to use a bit of gravity. Place a pillow under your bottom and this will naturally cause everything to retract into your body; this can make sex less uncomfortable and more enjoyable

Backache

I once had a patient who was suffering with backache; she'd had every test going looking for a slipped disc or some other cause; interestingly all her X-rays and MRI scans came back completely clear with no sign of a back problem. She had come to see me completely incidentally as she was suffering from stress incontinence. When I examined her I found the culprit straight away – she had a cystocele and a rectocele. She did lots of pelvic floor rehabilitation and some core strengthening exercises and sure enough her back pain went away. She was completely delighted, not only because she had got rid of her back pain (without having to have back surgery), but also because she'd fixed a prolapse she didn't even realize she had. So a great result all round.

Urinary Tract Infections

Urine infections are always a good reason to go to your doctor, as they can be very unpleasant and debilitating things. Usually a urine sample and urine test is required but if you don't usually suffer from urine infections, it's not a bad idea to ask your doctor to give you a vaginal examination to check whether a bladder prolapse (cystocele) is the cause of the infection. At the same time a bladder scan could be performed to see if you are emptying your bladder properly.

Sometimes with a cystocele urine pools in the prolapse and sits there stagnating until it becomes infected. If you are not emptying your bladder properly this can become a vicious circle; it's so important that you don't spend years going from one antibiotic to another when treating your prolapse was all that was needed to stop the infections happening. That's why you should always try and empty your bladder as best you can while you have your prolapse, using a technique called double voiding (see page 23).

Grades of Prolapse

Prolapse is often graded using an assessment tool called POP-Q (pelvic organ prolapse quantification system). This is the grading that your doctor or gynaecologist may use.

Grade 1

You may not even realize that you have a prolapse at this stage. It might be that following a routine smear test or other vaginal examination your doctor or nurse notices that you have a small prolapse and asks whether you feel like your pelvic floor is weak. If this is the case then treat this as a wake-up call to get on and do some pelvic floor rehabilitation as soon as possible. I have seen so many women over the years who have been jogging along through life with this little time bomb waiting to go off. Then suddenly something happens like a bad cough, the menopause or lifting a rather heavy toddler and what was a tiny prolapse suddenly becomes much worse. Having a small weakness in your pelvic floor and not being aware of it is completely normal, so please start your pelvic floor exercises today before it's too late.

Grade 2

This is when your bladder or bowel falls down far enough to be at the opening to the vagina. At this point it is more likely that you will be experiencing some or all of the symptoms of prolapse listed above.

Grade 3

This is when the pelvic organs begin to bulge out of the vaginal opening. It may feel really uncomfortable or painful.

Grade 4

This is the most severe form of prolapse and is when your entire bladder or uterus comes out of your vagina. Thankfully it is also the least common, as women will usually have sought help before it reaches this point. However, prolapse is still an under-reported problem so it's always important to seek help as soon as you can so your prolapse doesn't get worse.

The Main Causes of Prolapse
Childbirth
Childbirth itself is the most common cause of prolapse. A prolapse can happen following childbirth whatever type of delivery you have had, but it is more likely to happen if you had a long and difficult birth or if you had an assisted or operative (forceps or ventouse) vaginal delivery. Having large babies, or indeed having lots of babies, can increase the risk of having a prolapse.

A patient of mine had recently gone back to work following the very traumatic delivery of her first baby. She had suffered a second-degree tear and a grade 2–3 cystocele (see page 54). She worked really hard on her pelvic floor rehabilitation using electrical stimulation and the Squeezy app. As a result she is much better. She feels that at this point in her life her prolapse is manageable and because she has not finished her family she will probably have another baby within the next couple of years. So for now she will stay as she is and review what to do after her family is complete. Interestingly, now that she is back at her sedentary office-based job, she is even better as she is not spending all day lifting a heavy toddler!

However, a prolapse can happen sometimes even when you have a Caesarean, as just being pregnant and carrying a baby for nine months causes stresses and strains on your pelvic floor, so it's really important to pay attention to your pelvic floor even if you haven't had a vaginal delivery.

There is some evidence to suggest that age is relevant and being over thirty-five at the time of your first delivery could be a factor. So if you are starting your family in your thirties or older it's even more important to make sure that you have strong pelvic floor muscles prior to getting pregnant.

Constipation
I ask every single one of my patients whether they suffer with constipation and at least 50 per cent of them tell me yes, or at

least sometimes yes. That 'sometimes' is important; even occasional constipation is enough to turn a grade 1 prolapse into a grade 3 prolapse. So please, please refer to Chapter 9 to take action when it comes to your bowels.

Hysterectomy

It may seem odd to think that a hysterectomy could cause a prolapse to happen but it can. When you have had your uterus removed there is a 10–15 per cent risk of a vaginal vault prolapse in the future. So if you have had a hysterectomy and haven't done any post-operative pelvic floor rehabilitation I beg you to start today.

The Menopause

When you reach the menopause your oestrogen levels drop and your vaginal tissue becomes less elastic. Everything becomes more fragile and definitely more prone to a prolapse occurring. Your pelvic floor organs (bladder, bowel and uterus), which were just about hanging on in there, may drop and cause prolapse. Take a look at Chapter 7 for more information on pelvic floor issues during the menopause.

Heavy Lifting

It always amazes me when I ask my patients what they do. One of my prolapse patients was a PA to a very busy barrister. We were discussing her lifestyle and deciding what treatment would best help her recover. I had foolishly assumed that she had a relatively sedentary office job; not a bit of it! As her boss was a barrister he had massive files for all his cases and she was regularly lugging them around the office and to court. Her poor pelvic floor! When she realized the damage she was doing with all her heavy lifting she ordered a trolley and started to wheel the files about the office. She also enlisted the help of one of the juniors to help her on court days. It was a simple solution, but very effective. In this case there would have been very little point in her working super-hard on her pelvic floor rehabilitation only to undo all the good work every day at the office.

Weight Gain

For women aged fifty-five to sixty-five, weight gain is a major health concern. This is understandable as obesity is one of the most common nutrition-related disorders globally, and its prevalence is increasing. Worldwide, the prevalence of obesity has more than doubled since 1980. In 2008, 1.5 billion adults over the age of twenty were classed as overweight, based on their body mass index (BMI) and the studies show that there is a higher prevalence in women.[12]

I have a patient in her mid-fifties who is quite overweight and suffering from a grade 2 prolapse. She was ashamed of her weight and knew that things weren't right but wasn't yet able to face it. She went to her gynaecologist for a routine check-up and was told that her prolapse was much worse than the previous year and she absolutely must do something about it before the only option left was surgery. It still took her three months to make an appointment to see me but now she is on a mission to lose the weight and fix her pelvic floor.

I seem to spend my life telling people to lose weight and in general there is often a taboo about raising this concern directly. However, it's so important to try to maintain a healthy weight throughout your life so please don't resort to buying loose clothing to cover up weight gain. Sometimes it takes an unflattering photograph at a family wedding or on holiday to reveal the truth about the weight you have gained. Instead of putting the photo in the bin put it on the fridge door – anywhere that will motivate you to make a change now.

Excessive Coughing

This could be from asthma or smoking. The asthma you can't do very much about except to make sure you are managing it the best you can. On the other hand, smoking is something that you *can* do something about. There is a huge amount of information and support available to help you quit so I urge you to make the change now, not least because it will benefit your health more generally. If you need help a good place to start is by looking for help online, particularly at the charities QUIT and ASH (see Helpful Organizations, page 155).

Fibroids

Fibroids are benign growths found on the inside and the outside of your uterus and are very common. They can vary in size and you often don't know you have them unless they are giving you problems, for example heavy or painful periods, bleeding between periods, needing to pee frequently, lower back pain and sometimes pain during sex. They are sometimes picked up when you have a scan or a gynaecological examination. If you have very large and heavy fibroids (they can grow as big as a grapefruit) these can be heavy enough to cause a prolapse to happen.

Age

There is nothing we can do about getting older, apart from looking after ourselves as best we can. Life expectancy is increasing so we are living longer and being much more active. As we age there is an increased risk of vaginal prolapse but if we take care of our bodies we can enjoy a happy and healthy old age. Even if you are eighty years old it's still important to have a strong pelvic floor. You will hopefully live a lot longer than your granny did, so get started at once.

Number of Children

It appears that your risk of prolapse increases the more children you have. This is certainly not the only determining factor but it does make it even more important to ensure pelvic floor exercises are part of your routine.

A Hereditary Element

There is some evidence to suggest that prolapse is hereditary and on a few occasions in my career I have treated three generations of the same family. So if your mother had a prolapse it is especially important to start pelvic floor rehabilitation at whatever age you are at the moment. But all prolapses certainly are not hereditary so don't just think that because your mother didn't have a prolapse you are immune.

Hypermobility

Ehlers-Danlos syndrome or Marfans syndrome are rare forms of hypermobility. Hypermobility means that your joints are more flexible than normal so if you have either of these conditions you have a higher risk of both urinary incontinence and pelvic organ prolapse. It is also thought that prolapse is more common in women with hypermobility.[13] For more information contact the Hypermobility Syndromes Association (HMSA, see Helpful Organizations, page 155).

As you can see, quite a few of the causes of prolapse do not involve having a baby. So please, if you have any of these other problems like constipation, being overweight or hypermobility, you need to take extra special care of your pelvic floor.

Treatment for Prolapse

There are a number of ways that a prolapse can be treated and many of them should be used alongside each other.

Pelvic Floor Rehabilitation

The first line of treatment for pelvic organ prolapse has to be pelvic floor rehabilitation. So if you know that you have a prolapse do refer back to Chapter 2 to find the most relevant treatment for you. It is possible that if you have prolapse, you also have occasional stress or urge incontinence so rehabilitation will improve these symptoms too.

Vaginal pessaries are discussed in detail in Chapter 2. They can be extremely important and empowering in helping women with vaginal prolapse, although they can be used at any time during your life. You can use them for short periods or as long as you like, and they can easily be put in and taken out, so you can just wear them for sport or important events.

Lifestyle
As well as making pelvic floor exercises part of your daily routine there are other lifestyle changes you can make. Make sure that you do not become constipated by eating a healthy diet with plenty of vegetables and fibre, maintain a healthy weight, avoid lifting heavy things and if you smoke, try to give up.

If you have recently had a baby please don't put yourself under pressure to spring back to your pre-pregnancy shape – ignore the skinny bikini-clad celebrities featured in glossy magazines after recently giving birth to their third baby. I see lots of postnatal patients who have rushed back to jogging, often when they are still breastfeeding with low oestrogen levels; no surprise then that they start to experience vaginal heaviness. So please hang up your trainers for a while and avoid any high-impact activity until you are recovered enough from giving birth.

Surgery – Pelvic Floor Repair
Regardless of whether you do end up taking this route it is important to make sure that you try other options first, particularly pelvic floor rehabilitation. This will mean that your pelvic floor muscles are in as good a shape as they can be prior to surgery and this will help you recover. One thing that is for certain, surgery may correct your prolapse but it won't strengthen your pelvic floor muscles. Most gynaecologists and women's health specialists will recommend that you try pelvic floor rehabilitation and other treatments (see above) before offering surgery as a solution, if only so that you get into some good habits.

In general, surgery is rarely done until you are certain that you have finished having children as a further pregnancy may cause the prolapse to recur, taking you back to square one. Surgery may also not be a good idea if you have other serious health problems. Remember, a prolapse may not be a pleasant thing to have but it is not a life-threatening condition so if there are other ways of managing it conservatively it's always best to explore those first.

Surgery is performed either vaginally or laparoscopically under general anaesthetic. The aim is to repair the prolapse and ensure that your bladder and bowels are working normally afterwards. It usually requires a stay of at least one or two nights in hospital and a period of post-operative recovery. You are generally advised not to drive or lift anything for a few weeks and it's usually six weeks before you can resume normal activities such as exercise and sexual intercourse. This is definitely something to consider if you need to return to work or have young children, as there's no point having surgery if you don't allow yourself the time to recover.

As we have said, surgery may cure your prolapse but it will not make your pelvic floor stronger so please keep up a good pelvic floor exercise programme. You also have to remember that after your surgery there is always a small chance that where you didn't have stress incontinence before you do now, so you could be exchanging one problem for another. You could try wearing a vaginal pessary as a trial if you are planning to have surgery. Wearing the pessary returns your anatomy to a more normal shape and will hopefully tell you if you are about to swap one problem for another.

All these things would have to be discussed with your doctor prior to having an operation, to decide what is the best surgery for you.

I had one patient who did opt for surgery to repair her prolapse; she had had five large babies so unsurprisingly her pelvic floor had suffered rather a lot. She told me that when it came to having the surgery she became very anxious – even though she had done lots of preoperative pelvic floor rehabilitation with me before the operation – as, in her words, 'it was such an intimate place'. The great news is that she is very happy with the surgical result and feels back to her old self. Her sex life is good, she has no urinary problems and she is so delighted that her vagina and perineum all feel so much better, as she described it: 'nearly how it used to be before babies'. She has promised me that she will keep doing her pelvic floor exercises every day!

SIX

Pregnancy, Childbirth and the Pelvic Floor

Around 353,000 babies are born in the world every day, that's about 250 babies a minute. So that's a lot of pelvic floors to rehabilitate. In this chapter I will take you through the things that affect the pelvic floor during your pregnancy, the birth of your baby and then during the postnatal period – the time when your brain has turned to mush and you are not sure which way is up but most likely when problems arise. So my advice is to prepare yourself before and during pregnancy; it will be so much easier to restore your pelvic floor muscles to normal if you have taken the time to understand how they work before you give birth or, better still, before you even become pregnant.

The Royal College of Midwives reports that a third of existing and expectant mothers don't do pelvic floor exercises, despite their reported benefits. An online survey of 1,000 women in the UK revealed that 29.2 per cent who have had or are expecting a baby admitted to never practising the exercises. Much as I find it heartening that the other 70 per cent had at least done a few, it is concerning that nearly a third of women hadn't.

One country which definitely is more proactive in terms of addressing this issue is France, where intensive postnatal pelvic floor rehabilitation is the norm. Over the years I have had many

French women as patients. They often come with a 'prescription' from their doctor prescribing ten sessions of electrical stimulation, pelvic floor exercises and biofeedback training. I am always thrilled as they are highly motivated to getting their whole bodies back into shape after giving birth – not just their figure but their pelvic floor too.

It should be the same for us all but somehow it isn't. Imagine having a better sex life, not having stress incontinence or wetting your pants and just feeling generally better about yourself. How wonderful for your self-esteem, your future health and life in general.

Having a baby is one of the most special and amazing times of your life. It's a natural process, not an illness, but nevertheless your body goes through a massive upheaval. I have no doubt most of you went to some antenatal classes or are just about to, so I'm sure pelvic floor exercises will feature somewhere along the way. This is a brave new world of motherhood that you are entering or have entered and it's so important that your pelvic floor is not at the bottom of the list of things to deal with.

Historically babies have been delivered by women; midwifery is probably the oldest female profession. The role of the midwife is to help women through the whole process of childbirth and is incredibly important. Throughout history and up until about a hundred years ago everyone gave birth at home, attended by a midwife or birthing attendant. It was only with the advent of modern medicine that women started having babies in hospital. It's wonderful that now women have the choice to give birth in hospital with a midwife or an obstetrician, to have a home birth, to use a birthing pool and to have the sometimes necessary option of a Caesarean. Whichever way your baby is born you need to care for your pelvic floor.

Your pregnancy, birth and the following postnatal period all have an effect on your pelvic floor. By looking after it the best you can you will be for ever happy that you did.

Pregnancy and the Pelvic Floor

Finding out that you are pregnant is so exciting and probably the last thing on your mind is your pelvic floor or your bladder. Why would it be? For most of you it has probably behaved pretty well up to now. You may have leaked with a hearty laugh, maybe had giggle incontinence when you were a teenager, the occasional damp patch in your knickers or been bursting for the toilet on the odd occasion. But hey, that's normal, isn't it? And if it has only happened once or very rarely, why worry?

We know that you may have had the odd leak before you became pregnant or it's possible you thought that only happened to older women. During pregnancy and particularly in the second and third trimester you may start to suffer with stress incontinence. For some of you the problem will go away once your baby is born and may only come back if you become pregnant again or possibly when you reach the menopause. It doesn't mean that because you were lucky and your stress incontinence went away that you should not do your pelvic floor muscle training.[14]

A study carried out last year looked at thirty-eight trials done in twenty different countries involving 9,892 women. They concluded that if women in the early stages of pregnancy were given good advice about doing targeted pelvic floor exercises it could prevent the onset of urinary incontinence in the later stages of pregnancy and after you have given birth.[15] So the message here is that you should start doing your exercises straight away, even if the benefits are not felt until later on or even later in life.

Hopefully after reading this you will be better equipped to know what to expect and be able to understand and plan for after your baby is born. During pregnancy all sorts of changes happen to your body – hormonal changes, your growing uterus and general weight gain may have a part to play in troublesome incontinence now or later on in life.

Pregnancy usually lasts about forty weeks or nine months and is split up into three separate sections called trimesters.

The First Trimester (Week 1 to 12)
As you may know, morning sickness or nausea is a common symptom in early pregnancy. It may have been the first sign that you thought you might be pregnant. Vomiting can make you wet your knickers so starting your pelvic floor exercises the day that you find out you are pregnant is a very good idea – that is if you haven't already been doing them. Even at this early stage you may also find that you are peeing more often.

The Second Trimester (Week 13 to 26)
Hopefully the early symptoms of pregnancy (extreme tiredness and morning sickness) should start to disappear and you may be feeling better. You should have more energy and start to do a bit more exercise. However, this is also the point in the process when you might start having constipation. So please keep an eye out for it and make sure you deal with it right away (see Chapter 9).

The Third Trimester (Week 27 to the Birth of Your Baby)
Your growing size may make you feel increasingly tired at this point so it's really important to listen to your body and rest. However, it's good to keep doing gentle exercise such as walking or swimming; if you have to jog, go gently, listen to your body, be careful and make sure to keep hydrated. At this time your baby is growing bigger and getting ready to be born. With the extra weight of your baby on your bladder, you may find that you are having some unexpected leaks of urine.

Work and Pregnancy
It's not uncommon for women to work right up until just before they are about to give birth. If this is you, try to have a short rest in the middle of the day to take the pressure off your pelvic floor. Most employers are much more clued up about their

responsibilities towards pregnant employees so don't be afraid to ask for what you need. Looking after yourself now is the best thing you can do, as soon you'll need all your strength for life with a new baby.

Exercise During Pregnancy

Most types of exercise are safe to do throughout your pregnancy. It is important to keep active and fit; this will help you throughout your pregnancy and you will recover more quickly afterwards. However, be more careful in the final trimester as there is an increased risk of stress incontinence, prolapse and diastasis recti (see page 79). The best exercises are swimming, using a stationary exercise bike or going for a brisk walk. As a rule of thumb, try not to do any exercises that leave you breathless, particularly towards the end of your pregnancy.

Nutrition and Weight Gain

You will obviously gain weight in pregnancy but be careful not to make pregnancy an excuse to eat too much. It's not good for you or the baby, is hard to get rid of later and can make stress incontinence worse. Most women gain about 10–12kg during their pregnancy. There are no hard and fast rules, so try to stick to the advice given to you by your midwife or doctor.

Constipation

Constipation is a common complaint in pregnancy and affects many pregnant women. It is possibly caused by the increased level of progesterone in your body, which has the effect of slowing your bowels down.[16] It's important to discuss this here as unreported constipation during pregnancy can lead to pelvic floor dysfunction as well as distress. Please don't strain on the toilet thinking that everything is OK. It isn't, and you must sort it out straight away so please talk to your midwife or doctor about how best to deal with it. All that straining is like having a mini birth every day, so think of your poor pelvic floor!

Pelvic Girdle Pain

Pelvic girdle pain or symphysis pubis pain happens to some women during pregnancy. It causes discomfort that can be mild or severe in nature. It can be painful climbing the stairs, turning over in bed or even just when walking. If this is happening to you, you need to see a specialist physiotherapist as soon as possible to minimize the pain that you are in and start managing the problem in the best way that you can. Pelvic floor exercises may help so I hope you are already doing yours!

Childbirth and the Pelvic Floor

This section looks at types of childbirth and how they affect your pelvic floor muscles, including normal vaginal delivery, vaginal delivery with medical assistance (operative vaginal delivery) and Caesarean.

Vaginal Delivery

Delivering your baby vaginally is one of the most natural and wonderful things in the world – few things in life are more exciting or precious. However, it doesn't always come without consequences.

We all know that our vaginas are designed to give birth to babies, and they do so every day all over the world. However, damage to your pelvic floor muscles and your perineum (the area between your vagina and your anus) while giving birth is common. This damage can take the form of tears, episiotomies (a surgical cut at the opening of the vagina) or general stretching of the muscles. It's impossible to predict what will happen at the moment of delivery and there are so many variable factors. Did you have an epidural? How big is your baby? Is it your first, second or third child? Are you over thirty-five?

Perineal trauma affects around 85 per cent of women who have a vaginal birth in the UK each year and millions more worldwide.[17] The most common reasons for trauma are a baby weighing over 4kg, if it's your first baby, a long second or pushing stage of labour that lasts more than one hour, instrumental delivery (see below) and a baby that is in a posterior presentation (when the baby is facing your tummy instead of your spine). Many women will require some stitches after a vaginal delivery.

Ventouse (Vacuum-Assisted Extraction) or Forceps Delivery

You may need to have a ventouse or a forceps delivery if your midwife or doctor is concerned about your or your baby's health, if your labour isn't progressing as it should or if you are struggling to push adequately. This will occur in 10–12 per cent of vaginal deliveries in the UK. Following a ventouse or forceps delivery there is a chance that the perineal trauma suffered may be slightly worse than with a non-instrumental vaginal delivery. So it's even more important to start an intensive programme of pelvic floor rehabilitation after the birth of your baby.

Ventouse

A ventouse delivery involves placing a hard or soft metal or plastic cup on your baby's head, following which suction is applied. When you have a contraction you will be asked to push and your midwife or obstetrician will gently pull. This may have to be done a few times until your baby is born.

Forceps

Forceps look like a pair of curved tongs or spoons that fit around your baby's head. They come in two parts and are gently placed inside your vagina, one on either side of your baby's head. They are then locked together. As with the ventouse extraction, when you have a contraction you will be asked to push and your midwife or obstetrician will pull gently to deliver your baby. Again more than one pull may be needed.

At this point I would like to share with you an email from a patient of mine's husband that he sent to his co-workers after the forceps delivery of his son:

My wife was an ABSOLUTE rock star during delivery. Women are exponentially stronger than men. Giving birth to another human being is an unassailable argument and men are fortunate to be allowed to occupy the same planet as women.

Vaginal Tears

Vaginal tears are common when you have a vaginal delivery. A tear happens when your baby stretches your vagina during delivery, to the point where your skin tears. Your midwife or doctor will do their best to help you avoid a tear during labour. The idea is to let your baby's head be born slowly and gently. This gives the skin and muscles of the perineum time to stretch and hopefully without tearing.

There is evidence to suggest that performing perineal massage in the last few weeks of pregnancy (from about thirty-four weeks) can help prevent tearing during the delivery of your baby. This is particularly of benefit with your first baby. There are various ways of doing this but one way is to lie on your bed, ideally after a bath or shower when your blood vessels are dilated and you are hopefully nice and relaxed. If you wish, your husband or partner can help you. You'll need some unscented neutral oil, preferably organic, or you can use unscented lubricating gel if you prefer (you can buy these in pharmacies). Apply to your fingers and start to massage your perineum (the bit between your vagina and anus). You can then insert one or two fingers into your vagina and apply a downward pressure towards your anus, moving your fingers from side to side in a 'U' movement. Try to do this for a few minutes as often as you like, ideally every day or every other day.[18]

If a tear does happen to you they are graded into the following degrees of severity:

- A first-degree tear affects the skin of your perineum and/or your labia and usually requires little intervention.

- A second-degree tear causes injury to your perineum and perineal muscles, but not your anal sphincter. This type of tear will usually need stitches.
- A third-degree tear is injury to the skin and muscle of your perineum as well as part of your anal sphincter.
- A fourth-degree tear is when the tear extends into your anus or rectum.

Episiotomy

An episiotomy is a surgical cut made by either your doctor or midwife. It's a cut in the perineum between the vagina and the anus and is usually done if your baby urgently needs to be delivered quickly or if forceps or ventouse are going to be used. It may also be done if there is a risk of a severe vaginal tear. An episiotomy will have to be stitched afterwards.

Caesarean Section

A Caesarean is much less traumatic to the pelvic floor than a vaginal delivery. But the process of pregnancy and the weight of your unborn baby all have a part to play, regardless of the method of delivery. Multiple pregnancies will also put more pressure on your pelvic floor muscles. So don't think that if you are having a caesarean then you can get away with not doing your exercises!

Women who have had a really traumatic first childbirth often ask me whether they should consider a Caesarean the second time around. This is a very difficult question to answer and varies hugely from person to person. In general, if you have a normal vaginal delivery second time round you will not exacerbate the problems caused by the first birth, although if you have several babies then your pelvic floor will start to suffer further. So a Caesarean isn't necessarily the answer; it just means you really need to work hard on recovering pelvic floor strength. However, for anyone who has faecal urgency, faecal leakage or the inability to control wind, I personally would always recommend a Caesarean with further pregnancies, as if these problems become worse they are often extremely hard to sort out with exercises or even surgery.

The Postnatal Period

Surprisingly little attention is devoted to recuperation of the pelvic floor – unless you live in France or have suffered a third- or fourth-degree tear. Why? I could weep for the amount of times I have heard women say, 'I think I may have been given a leaflet but it's a long time ago,' or, 'I feel so bad – I know I should have been doing my pelvic floor exercises at the bus stop.'

Largely gone is the life that my mother led when she was bringing up me and my brother. Every day (and she is still doing it aged eighty-two) she eats her lunch then puts her feet up for half an hour on the sofa for a snooze. While that might not seem realistic or possible for you it's so important to be kind to yourself and allow time to rest after you've had a baby, as it will be of huge benefit in the long term. I see lots of patients who are completely shocked to discover that they have postnatal prolapse; they have started running round the park just six weeks after giving birth and suddenly they have a heavy feeling in the vagina. Like most things there has to be a balance; certainly do keep fit, but be careful not to damage your pelvic floor. Just because you can't see it don't assume that it doesn't need attention.

Issues with Abdominal Muscles (Diastasis Recti)
Do you still look pregnant weeks (or even months) after giving birth? It may not be just that baby weight that you are trying desperately to get rid of; it could be down to the separation of your abdominal muscles that happens when you are pregnant.

When you are pregnant it's common for your abdominal muscles to separate as your baby gets larger inside you, due to your changing hormones. This tends to happen in the later stages of pregnancy as your uterus and baby grow. In general the separation will lessen in the first few months after giving birth but in some cases the muscles don't return to normal as quickly as they should.

Every single postnatal woman I see I check to see if their abdominal muscles are still separated. But it's relatively easy to check yourself and everyone who is reading this and who has had a baby (even if it was ages ago) should check. If you think that you have a division of the muscles it's important that you seek professional advice from a women's health physiotherapist.

How to Check Yourself

Lie down on your back with your knees bent and feet flat on the floor. Place the palm of your hand flat on your stomach near your tummy button and curl your fingers slightly so the tips of your fingers are flat on your tummy. Now slowly lift your head as though you are drawing your chin on to your chest. This action causes your rectus abdominis muscle to contract.

When you do this, if your fingertips find a gap that two of your fingertips can fit into between the muscles, then this is a diastasis. If the gap is four fingers wide this is a severe case of diastasis and surgery may be required. Always remember that if you do have surgery to correct this it won't improve your muscle tone, either of your rectus abdominis or your pelvic floor, so you should still work on improving muscle function.

While you are seeking help it's a good idea to avoid the following:

- Stomach crunches and sit-ups
- Sitting bolt upright when getting out of bed – try to roll out
- Carrying your baby (and certainly your toddler) on one hip
- Constipation and coughing unless you are supporting your abdominal muscles (do this by pulling your belly button in towards your spine)

Sometimes you will be given a support to wear. There are varying schools of thought on this as to whether it's helpful or not. I personally think if it makes you feel more comfortable and safer and your abdominal muscles are being protected then it's a good idea. However, you should still take good care of yourself (see above), even if you are wearing a supporting garment.

I remember a woman who came to see me with stress incontinence. She had had three children varying in age from six down to two. She asked me to check her stomach as it hadn't felt the same since having her children. Sure enough, she had a large division of her muscle and it had been left totally untreated. I gave her my advice on what not to do (it turns out she had always carried her young children on one hip). I then referred her to a specialist physiotherapist to see if her problem could be fixed with exercise alone. At last she is addressing the problem. She had no idea what was wrong; all she knew was that it wasn't like that before she had her children. She'd just assumed it was one of those things that you have to put up with – a consequence of having children. I have made sure that she now knows (as all of you reading this now do) that this is not normal and you need to do something about it. I am sure that there are lots of you out there who have been busily doing millions of sit-ups and stomach crunches in a bid to make your mummy tummy go away, little realizing that you could be making the problem worse instead of better.

Postnatal Sex
A study published by the *British Journal of Obstetrics and Gynaecology*[19] found that 83 per cent of women suffered sexual problems in the first three months after giving birth and only 15 per cent sought help. The study also found that 89 per cent of women had resumed sexual activity after six months. So if you are suffering please tell someone as it will probably make you feel better and there also may be a simple solution. There is no right answer for when you should have sex for the first time after giving birth

although the advice is generally to wait for 4–6 weeks, or at least until your postpartum bleeding has stopped.

There are some couples having sex after a couple of weeks and there are some who still aren't having sex months and months later. It's a brave new world you are dealing with; with sleepless nights, breastfeeding and a new baby to take care of you may just not fancy sex at all, while some of you may feel more sexy than you did before. It's a very personal thing.

I recently saw a woman who had been breastfeeding her baby for six months. She was very concerned that she and her husband had hardly had any sex since their baby had arrived. When I saw her, her pelvic floor tone was very poor and her vagina was dry due to lack of oestrogen caused by the breastfeeding. She worked very hard on her pelvic floor rehabilitation and came to see me during the process. What with the vaginal laxity and dryness that she was suffering from, sex was the last thing on her mind. However, once her pelvic floor muscles were stronger (this was achieved first with some electrical stimulation and then with the use of the Elvie trainer) she felt more like her old self. She also stopped breastfeeding around this time and had a period. One day she bounded in to see me full of *joie de vivre*; her sex life was back on track and she felt confident again. So don't worry if you don't feel like having fabulous sex when you have just had a baby. Do your exercises, take your time and things will come naturally.

Sex may be just how it was before you had your baby or it might not. Sometimes it's painful. It's possible that you have a prolapse and this can cause pain, particularly if your cervix is a bit lower than it used to be, or you've had stitches and the area still feels sore or tender.

Another reason why sex can be painful is that after giving birth your levels of oestrogen drop and this can lead to vaginal dryness – the last thing you need when you are just restarting your sex life! Even if you've never had to use it before buy some vaginal gel, lubricant or oil and use it the first time you have sex.

One word of caution: if you're rediscovering the joys of having sex again don't forget the contraception! I have done quite a few pregnancy tests in my clinic for women who come to see me saying, 'I have been great, my pelvic floor has felt back to normal and suddenly it feels really weak again. What do you think is happening?' Sure enough, a positive pregnancy test follows.

Please start your pelvic floor exercises now if you haven't already. Don't belong to that third of women who are not doing any exercises at all. The pelvic floor is an amazing structure and damage can undoubtedly be done to it during delivery. So now that you have read about what can happen to your pelvic floor during pregnancy and childbirth, take the time to get together with all your pregnant and new-mum friends – even those that haven't given childbirth a second thought yet – and get motivated and squeezing!

SEVEN

The Menopause and Beyond

The menopause, sometimes referred to as the climacteric by the medical profession (climacteric means 'a critical period or event') is something that happens to all women. Although it is a normal part of a woman's life, the symptoms it brings with it can feel far from normal and can send you plunging into a whole new world of stress incontinence, absent-mindedness, hot flushes and many other joyful, confusing or irritating things!

Menopause usually starts when you are in your late forties or early fifties but this can vary quite a lot. In relatively rare cases it can happen either earlier or later than this. If it happens before you are forty it is called the premature menopause. The Daisy Network is an organization that offers advice and support for those undergoing premature menopause (see Helpful Organizations, page 157).

As life expectancy is increasing women will, on average, spend about a third to half their lives going through some stage of the menopause (see below). It's very important that we are able to live this part of our lives to the maximum, not bogged down or defeated by the symptoms of the menopause. We need to understand what is happening to our bodies in order to be able to deal successfully with the consequences.

An estimated one billion women living in the world today have experienced the menopause.[20] This is a huge number of women when you consider that the world population is about 7.4 billion. We need to look after women in the menopause better – too many women just muddle on through. A recent report by the British Menopause Society found that half the women going through the menopause hadn't visited a doctor, as many were 'too embarrassed'.

The menopause is a time in your life when your body starts to produce less oestrogen. Your body's store of eggs is used up and your periods start to become irregular, eventually stopping altogether. Some women have hardly any menopausal symptoms and sail through this period of their lives barely realizing anything has happened, except perhaps noticing the lack of periods. But let's face it, after forty years of tampons, pads and period pains a lot of women could not be more delighted about this. However, for many women the menopause is a confusing, distressing and difficult time.

The menopause comes in three distinct phases:

- Perimenopause
- Menopause
- Post-menopause

Perimenopause
The oestrogen in your body isn't just there one day and gone the next. Like your store of eggs, oestrogen diminishes over time. This phase is called the perimenopause. It's a time of life that's endlessly discussed and worried over. Patients often say to me, 'Is this it?' as if the end of the world is nigh. The one thing that is for sure is that we are all affected differently by the menopause. I firmly believe that it can be a time to embrace life and enjoy every minute. If you have children they may have grown up, or at least are hopefully a little less needy. It's time for you to have some me

time, to have a bit of fun and do all those things that you have been putting off for years. Don't forget though that even though your periods are starting to become irregular, you can still become pregnant so do carry on taking precautions.

Menopause

When you haven't had a period for a year or so you are probably in the menopause. If you have a Mirena coil in situ, or you are on the pill, it's harder to tell what's happening as you may not have had a normal cycle for however long you have been using the coil or the pill. You can have a blood test to check your hormone levels, but it's not really necessary unless your doctor requests it. Don't forget that this is a natural process after all.

The symptoms of the menopause usually last for about 4 to 5 years. During this time the symptoms can remain intense or slowly diminish with time.

Post-menopause

This is when the symptoms of the menopause have diminished. It is a time to take care of yourself as other problems may occur such as osteoporosis and heart disease.

Pelvic Floor Problems and the Menopause

How many times have you seen a menopausal woman on a trampoline? Something I hear all the time is: 'I will never get on my granddaughter's trampoline again! I was shocked to find I had wet my pants. Help!' The trampoline and the skipping rope, for that matter, are the ultimate bladder challenges so if all your other bladder issues are better after you have followed my programme of pelvic floor rehabilitation then you may have to accept that your trampolining days are over.

I have said for years that I should ask everyone who comes to see me to put £1 in a charity box when they start a sentence with, 'Well, I had children in my thirties and everything has been fine, apart from the occasional leak with a bad cough – that's normal, isn't it? Now things are much worse: I can't get to the toilet in time and I have a horrible heavy feeling in my vagina like everything is going to fall out.' I would have raised a lot of money for charity over the years.

Stress Incontinence

You may have had a bit of stress incontinence over the last twenty or so years but if it wasn't bad enough to be wearing a pad I suspect you never got around to doing anything about it. Suddenly it's the menopause and things are much worse. Stress incontinence is discussed in much more detail in Chapter 3.

Frequency, Urgency and Urge Incontinence

The symptoms of frequency and urgency can be harder to deal with when your oestrogen levels are starting to drop, but don't panic: there are still things you can do to improve the situation. But if you are reading this in your thirties, take note: it's much easier to sort your pelvic floor out now while you still have all your oestrogen.

Due to the decrease in your oestrogen levels you can suddenly start having to run to the toilet. It might be after that double macchiato that you knew was a bad idea; it could be the sight of your front door at the end of a long busy day triggers an urgent need to pee, causing you to wince, cross your legs or hop up and down while you find your keys. You tell yourself it's ridiculous, you only went an hour ago. But your bladder is having none of it and if you don't get into the house fast disaster will strike.

On the other hand, this terrifying scenario of wetting your knickers on your doorstep is often the point when a lot of women realize they need to do something about it – I say this from all my years of experience. And that can only be a good thing.

Prolapse

If you are going through the menopause and don't have a prolapse or don't know that you have a prolapse (a lot of small ones give no symptoms) please start a pelvic floor rehabilitation programme as it may stop you from having a prolapse in the future. See Chapter 5 for more information on pelvic organ prolapse.

Atrophic Vaginitis and Vaginal Dryness

Atrophic vaginitis means that the walls of your vagina start to thin and lose some of their elasticity. It can be accompanied by vaginal dryness, pain during sex, urinary infections and itching and soreness of the vulva. This is due to your body having less oestrogen.

It would appear that women who have not had a vaginal delivery tend to suffer more from the symptoms listed above. This is entirely logical, as the vagina hasn't been stretched during a vaginal birth. Without vaginal delivery your vagina is smaller and tighter so it can become more difficult to have penetrative sex than if you have had four large babies delivered vaginally. On the other hand, multiple vaginal deliveries can cause women to suffer with vaginal laxity and unfulfilling sex for years. Both problems can be dealt with effectively.

All women can suffer from atrophic vaginitis. However, they are too often embarrassed to visit their doctor because things are not right 'down there'. Often they don't know why this is; they just know that sex is now super painful – often for days afterwards.

I had a lovely patient once who was very happily married and she and her husband had always enjoyed a good sex life. However, when she came to see me she had been having painful intercourse for about five years without saying anything to her husband, let alone her doctor. She didn't want to upset her husband and the longer she had left it, the more she realized how upset he would be to think she'd been in pain. As for visiting a doctor, she was just too shy. She eventually told her husband and started using vaginal oestrogen, pelvic floor rehabilitation and some vaginal dilation therapy. I'm glad to say things are now so much better.

Cystitis

Cystitis is an inflammation of your bladder usually caused by a urinary tract infection. Urinary tract infections are the most common bacterial infection in women in general and in postmenopausal women in particular.[21]

You may have suffered from urine infections all your life or they may have started happening at the beginning of your sexual life. Urine infections are more common in women as the female urethra is shorter (so bacteria have less far to travel) and much closer to the anus than it is in men. They could be caused by a cystocele (a prolapse of the bladder) or maybe by the thinning of the vaginal tissue. Whatever the reason it is not pleasant or particularly comfortable. The usual symptoms are a burning sensation when you pass urine, either cloudy or smelly urine or both, urgency and frequency to pass urine. Sometimes you may feel very unwell and have a high temperature and the shivers. Sometimes you may have lower back or abdominal pain as well.

I have treated lots of women who have started having recurrent urinary tract infections at the menopause (recurrent means having more than two infections in the last six months or three in a year). It can become a vicious cycle: have sex, get an infection, do a urine test, take antibiotics, get better, have sex again and then the whole cycle repeats itself. This type of recurrent urinary tract infection can occur at any age.

To help this problem make sure that you have a good fluid intake of at least 1.5 litres a day. Sometimes doctors will prescribe an antibiotic to be taken before sex or your doctor may give you a low-dose antibiotic to be taken over a few months to help get rid of all the bacteria causing the problem.

Other ways to treat recurrent cystitis are using vaginal oestrogen, improving your pelvic floor tone and trying to empty your bladder more effectively by using the double voiding technique (see page 23). Always pee before and after sex; this will 'rinse' any bacteria out of your urethra and is a good self-help technique.

Reduced Sex Drive

Reduced sex drive is something that can affect women going through the menopause; however, it is not always the case and in some women sex drive actually improves. There is the freedom from the worry of getting pregnant and the fear that small children will come rushing in when you are in the middle of the act is no more. No shared hotel rooms on holiday, or when staying with grandparents or friends. There may even be fewer financial pressures so you may have more money and time to enjoy life.

On the other hand you may just not fancy sex any more. It is possible that you still have teenagers to look after; in different ways they can be as needy as small children what with exam pressures, angst over their first love and all the other teenage things that we all went through. You may be caring for elderly parents and trying to work and juggle all these things is not conducive to feeling super sexy, particularly with that half a stone you seem to have gained and your plummeting oestrogen levels.

It's worth reminding ourselves that it's not just women who are getting a bit older. Your husband or partner is ageing too and may have prostate problems or high blood pressure or be taking medication that makes erections more difficult. As a couple you are ageing gently together and this is a normal part of life's cycle. The key is for both of you to find a happy place where your sex life sits. If that seems difficult there is very good help available, so do please read the next chapter for more information. If both of you do your pelvic floor exercises, you may be amazed at the results! If medication is required a visit to your doctor may sort things out quickly, while if it's counselling you need the Sexual Advice Association is the place to seek help (see Helpful Organizations, page 158).

Constipation

If you find that you are suffering from constipation then please read Chapter 9. This definitely needs dealing with as soon as you can as the thinning of your vaginal tissue during menopause can leave you much more vulnerable to having a prolapse.

Other Problems Associated with the Menopause

The menopause affects women in different ways; some will have relatively few symptoms while others might feel like they are struggling to feel normal. Many of these are not associated with the pelvic floor but can still be pretty debilitating.

Hot Flushes and Night Sweats

How often have you seen women fanning themselves on the train, bus or other crowded places? Believe me, it's not because it's 30 degrees outside! Oddly, hot flushes are sort of 'OK' to talk about, unlike pelvic floor collapse.

How many times a night are you turning your pillow over because it's drenched in sweat? If this is you, consider buying a cooling pad insert for your pillow. It goes really cold when you put your hot head on it, which is very soothing and frankly marvellous.

The most common symptom of the menopause is hot flushes, happening to about 75 per cent of women. I can tell you that I am never wearing a polo-neck jumper ever again. My mother-in-law once said to me as I was trying to fend off a hot flush, 'Never wear wool next to your skin.' It's good advice.

Insomnia

A friend of mine was plagued by insomnia; it was the only symptom she has ever had during the menopause. In this modern, fast-moving world that we live in, insomnia can be a disaster. With a very busy working and home life she became a gibbering wreck in a few short weeks. Help was at hand in the form of HRT gel. For her, this was the miracle cure and she no longer has insomnia. This is not for everyone and should be considered under the guidance of your doctor but if you are having any problems with the menopause do please find ways to address them so you can move on with your life, rather than just muddling through. I use my friend here as an example as her problem was so bad she thought that she was a danger driving and that she might fall asleep at the wheel. Whatever you do, don't ignore your problems, thinking that they will just go away.

Joint and Muscle Stiffness

This is caused by hormonal changes that happen at the menopause. You may be worse in the morning and get better as the day wears on. It's a good reason to stay active – lots of research shows that regular low-impact exercise such as swimming, cycling and yoga is good for bone strength as well as your general health. It's also your moment to give up smoking, a known risk factor for osteoporosis (decreased bone density and weak bones that are more likely to fracture).

Mood Swings

A former patient of mine, who I had seen about ten years previously after she'd had her children, made an appointment to see me. She was feeling very low, had depression-like symptoms and was cross all the time. She and her family were in despair and to cap it all, she discovered she'd had a prolapse. Although the prolapse was bothering her and she was very keen to work on improving it, her main worry was how she was feeling in herself. She had been using a Mirena coil (an intrauterine device) so hadn't been having much in the way of periods. She is a very busy lawyer with two teenagers so the menopause was not something she had even given a thought to. She didn't *feel* menopausal, nor was she struggling with hot flushes or night sweats, but I felt sure that the sudden feelings of prolapse and her mood changes were a definite sign.

She consulted her doctor and a blood test confirmed that she was very definitely menopausal. Her doctor suggested antidepressants to tackle her mood changes and depression (these can be of help to women during the menopause) but my patient insisted that she didn't need antidepressants; what she needed was HRT. She had never been depressed in her life and felt that the feelings she was having could only be related to the menopause. She started taking HRT and the next time she came to see me she told me that I had saved her life. She was totally back to her old self and able to run her busy life again. We are still working on strengthening her pelvic floor muscles but she is improving all the time and her prolapse is now manageable. It's always worth exploring what is the right medication for you, if you feel that medication is the way forward.

Memory Issues

Do you sometimes go upstairs and for the life of you can't remember what you went up to get? Did you see someone that you know really well across the street but you simply can't think of his or her name? Don't panic: it's not Alzheimer's and you are not going mad, it's most likely a symptom of the menopause. It is not fully understood why this happens but it may have something to do with your dropping oestrogen levels. It may simply be that if you are suffering from insomnia or night sweats you will naturally wake up tired and fuzzy-headed. Having a lot of hot flushes during the day can be draining and distracting.

Try to eat well and take some exercise and get some fresh air whenever you can. It's really important to keep yourself stimulated. You may already have a very busy taxing job on top of your home life but if not, take up something that will stimulate your brain, like learning a language or even writing a book!

Weight Gain

Are you suddenly a stone heavier than you have ever been? How did that happen? If your clothes are tight and you've put on weight, especially around your middle, your poor pelvic floor is going to be suffering the effects.

Obesity is a public health problem with overweight individuals representing about 20 per cent of the adult world population. Age is the main cause of weight gain in mid-life; from this time on average we increase in weight by about 0.5kg per year. However, hormonal changes across the perimenopause substantially contribute to increased central and abdominal fat and abdominal obesity.[22] So all you women reading this take heart that you haven't suddenly been sleepwalking to the biscuit tin in the middle of the night. It's your hormones that have been at it again.

Weight control has an essential role in menopausal health and should be considered early in the perimenopause to improve quality of life. Being overweight not only affects your pelvic floor but it impacts on your self-esteem and your general wellbeing. So you will need to work extra hard on maintaining a steady weight. It's so important and we all need a bit of encouragement. Start by doing really simple things like climbing an extra flight of stairs a day or maybe walking to the shops instead of taking the car. Some studies suggest that the use of hormone replacement therapy is not associated with increased weight and indicate that it might be helpful in the reduction of overall body fat.[23]

Ways to Tackle the Symptoms of the Menopause
As mentioned before, women will go through the menopause with very different experiences, with some having just one or two of the above symptoms. Whatever it is you are going through, the advice below will be useful to all menopausal women as there is no one quick fix that will solve all your problems.

Pelvic Floor Rehabilitation
Hopefully by now you will have realized how important it is to maintain a strong pelvic floor. Please refer to Chapter 2 for the ultimate guide to pelvic floor strength.

Lifestyle Changes

Cutting down the amount of caffeine and alcohol you drink may help reduce hot flushes, as well as improve your memory and reduce urinary frequency and urgency. Taking a moderate amount of exercise is always a good idea; think swimming, cycling and yoga – not trampolining! Always eat a healthy balanced diet with plenty of vegetables and fibre to avoid becoming constipated.

For all of us living life at a frenetic pace the menopause is a time to start caring for yourself a bit more. By this I don't mean just the physical things like diet and exercise, it's important to care for our minds too. Treat yourself to a lovely hot bath with candles and gentle music, or a luxurious massage or facial. You will feel more relaxed, even if it doesn't rid you of the immediate symptoms of the menopause. Maybe you would benefit from doing a mindfulness or meditation programme (see Helpful Organizations, page 155). There are also lots of alternative therapies available such as acupuncture, which has been shown to help with the symptoms of the menopause.[24]

Vaginal Oestrogen

I am a huge fan of vaginal oestrogen. It has given many women their sex lives back and is so easy to use. If you have a dry or possibly sore vagina then do see your doctor, as vaginal oestrogen could be the solution to your problems. Lack of vaginal oestrogen is a very under-reported problem. It can be embarrassing to tell your doctor that sex is painful, that you are struggling to get to the toilet in time, but it's very possible that vaginal oestrogen can improve things, even an irritable bladder.

Vaginal oestrogen comes in various forms and it is always prescribed and monitored by your doctor.

- **Vagifem pessaries or vaginal inserts** These are inserted into your vagina, giving you a small dose of something called estradiol (similar to the oestrogen that your body used to make). You normally start by using the pessaries every day for two weeks and then you move on to a maintenance dose of twice a week.

- **Estring** This is a soft, flexible vaginal ring that emits estradiol. It is positioned inside your vagina and remains in place for about three months. You may be taught how to change it yourself or, if you prefer, your doctor or healthcare practitioner can change it for you. It can be worn during sex but can be removed if you prefer – just rinse it in lukewarm water and don't forget to put it back in afterwards.
- **Oestrogen creams** A cream with the active ingredient estriol is inserted into the vagina using an applicator. You usually start with a certain daily dose over a period of between one and three weeks before dropping to a reduced dose twice a week.

Vaginal oestrogen is sometimes used prior to surgery for prolapse so if you are having an operation to repair a prolapse do check whether vaginal oestrogen therapy would be good to use before and after your operation.

If you have symptoms of vaginal dryness and are not keen on taking or can't take hormone replacement therapy, vaginal oestrogen may be an option for you and you should speak to your doctor.

Even if you are using vaginal oestrogen you will probably need to use a vaginal lubricant as well when you are having sex. There are now a variety of good-quality lubricants on the market. They can be gel- or oil-based so do try different ones to see which one is the best for you and your partner.

Vaginal Dilators
If you are not having sex because of pain and vaginal dryness, it can be difficult to address. It may have started to happen slowly over a period of time as your oestrogen levels start to fall. Vaginal

dilator therapy is a gentle self-treatment that is easy to do and can be extremely beneficial to your sex life. Using vaginal dilators is a great way of gently stretching the vaginal tissue and giving you confidence.

Vaginal dilators come in a set of five – you start by inserting the smallest one into your vagina using lots of lubrication; it sometimes helps to contract your pelvic floor muscles around it while the dilator is inside you. This is good for your pelvic floor muscles and will help you get used to using the dilators. It helps to keep the dilator in place for a few minutes, gently pushing it back and forth. Carry on using the dilators until you have used the one that is as big or a bit bigger than your husband or partner's penis. Find a time to do this when you know you won't be disturbed as you won't be looking at your most glam! It can be a really wonderful treatment if you have all but given up on your sex life due to pain and discomfort. You should try to do the therapy every day or at least every other day. Some women may decide to do this with their partner as a form of foreplay but it is up to you as a couple to decide.

Hormone Replacement Therapy
This is a book in itself and many have been written on the subject. I am not an expert in HRT, nor will I try to be here, but I will outline the different types of hormone replacement therapy to hopefully give you a starting point if this is something that you are considering.

Hormone replacement therapy has been studied widely across the world; according to the Royal College of Obstetricians and Gynaecologists, HRT works and is safe for most women. There was much controversy in the media regarding HRT in the late 1990s and early 2000s as a result of two large studies, which raised concerns over the use of HRT. This led to a massive reduction in women taking HRT and a general reluctance of doctors to prescribe it.

At the moment there are lots of recent and ongoing trials that seem to have much more favourable results. A good place to read about HRT is on the Women's Health Concern website; this is the patient arm of the British Menopause Society. You can then decide with your doctor, gynaecologist or menopause specialist if it is an appropriate treatment for you. If you start taking HRT you should have a proper annual review with your doctor.

Hormone replacement therapy is used for treating the symptoms of the menopause. It is usually prescribed in the lowest possible dose that relieves your symptoms. The main hormonal medications involved are oestrogens and progesterones. If you have not had a hysterectomy you will need to take progesterone as well as oestrogen because with oestrogen alone the lining of your womb may grow excessively, leading to a possible increased risk of endometrial cancer.

HRT comes as a tablet, a gel or a patch. The tablets are taken daily and the gel is rubbed into your skin each day. The patches are normally changed twice a week.

Bioidentical hormones can be prescribed by some doctors. You should discuss their use very carefully with your doctor, and take only the hormone therapies that are regulated and approved, as some of them don't have the scientific evidence that they are safe or effective.

Then there are over-the-counter herbal remedies. As with any herbal remedies it's sensible to check with your doctor or pharmacist before taking them so you know they are not going to interfere with any other medication you are taking.

I hope this chapter has given you a better understanding of what can happen during and after the menopause and made you realize that there are lots of other people out there like you – one billion women in fact! You don't have to put up with any symptoms that are bothering you just because your mother did – there is help out there!

EIGHT

Sex and the Pelvic Floor

Our pelvic floor muscles are very important for sex so if you haven't been motivated to start your pelvic floor exercises by now, this is the time to take note of the benefits! Doing the exercises covered in Chapter 2 helps increase the blood supply to the vagina and penis, improves muscle tone and helps maintain nerve activity, resulting in improved sexual sensation and satisfaction. Like any exercise regime, if you have strong muscles you feel good about yourself. I am sure we have all felt boosted by a long walk or a great workout. The same is true for your vagina or your penis, resulting in better erections, which (pardon the pun!) is all very uplifting.

Sex is something that we have all been doing for ever – none of us would be here without it! However, habits and trends change over time as our lifestyles change. A study published in *The Lancet* based on a national survey of sexual attitudes over thirty years found that we are starting to have sex for the first time younger than ever before, and we are carrying on having sex much later on in life. It also found that we are having sex slightly less often than we used to due to fewer people being married or living together (as there is less opportunity).[25] We all vary hugely in how often we want to have sex and despite the fact that talking about sex is less of a taboo and it's far more visible on television and social media, we are still not very open about it.

If you need help with understanding how your pelvic floor plays a part in your sexual health then what you are about to read should give you a good insight into this part of your body.

Women and Sex

I think that one of the main reasons why women tend to ignore their pelvic floor is that we don't often look at our genitals, particularly if they are not giving us any trouble. It's possible that you had a look with a mirror as a teenager trying to insert your first ever tampon. Or possibly out of curiosity after having had a baby? In my experience most people rarely look down under at their vulva and vagina. Since I have been writing this book, I have been asking my postnatal patients if they have 'had a look'; most of them said that they had not. Fear of what they might see might be the reason, or it may just be a case of 'out of sight, out of mind'. Some women have a little look if they are sore or worried about a prolapse and even then not as many as you might expect. In my experience younger women tend to be a bit better at knowing their anatomy and are more likely to have had a peek just to see that it all looks reassuringly as they think it should. I have been asked so many times by worried young women, 'Is my labia normal? I think it is so ugly.' I say to everyone: love your labia and embrace your beautiful body. Thank goodness we are all quite unique so please don't be seduced by social media and pictures of what is passed off as perfectly shaped – everyone is and we should all be different.

It's important as women that we understand the anatomy of our vulva and our vagina, so let's all get better acquainted with our bits! A great place to start is to get a small hand mirror and take a look.

The Vulva

It is a common misconception that the vulva is the vagina. In fact, it's everything you can see on the outside. It is made up of:

- **Mons pubis or pubic mound** This is the rounded mound which covers the pubic bone. It is sometimes called the mound of Venus as it acts a bit like a cushion during sex.
- **Labia majora or outer labia (lips)** The outer lips of your labia look like the rest of your skin. This area and the mons pubis are where your pubic hair grows.
- **Labia minora or inner labia (lips)** The skin of the inner labia is a different colour, which varies from pink to brown depending on your skin colour. This area of your body has a lot of nerve endings and it enjoys being touched. Before puberty the inner lips are hidden away inside the outer lips. As we develop the inner labia grows bigger. In some women it stays tucked away inside the

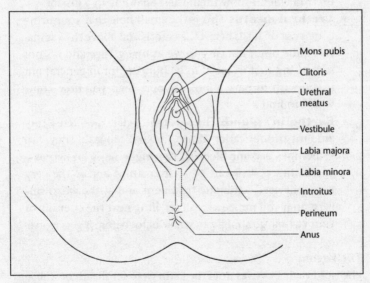

Vulva

outer lips, while in other women one or both of the labia minora protrude out, but both ways are totally normal. I worry about the growing trend for cosmetic surgery in the form of labioplasty, a surgical procedure to reduce the size of the labia minora. In my entire career I have only ever had one patient who genuinely needed this procedure. She had a very small frame with very large inner labia so it was impossible for her to wear a bikini, and trousers were very uncomfortable and often caused chafing. She went ahead and had the surgery and it was a big success.

- **The vestibule or introitus** This is the part that surrounds the vaginal and urethral opening. Think of it as the entrance to the vagina.
- **Clitoris** Your clitoris is a source of sexual pleasure and is visible externally as a pea-sized nub located above your urethra. It is *not* where urine comes out, despite what many people think; I have seen many women point to it as their urethra when I show them their anatomy in a mirror.
- **Urethral meatus** This is the small hole that your urine comes out of. It sits below the clitoris and above the vagina. It is quite often not easy to see at first glance and it's not something that we need to go hunting for in general but if you wish to have a look at yours then you now know where to find it!
- **Bartholin's glands** The Bartholin's glands excrete a tiny amount of lubrication during sexual arousal. They can sometimes become blocked, causing what is known as a Bartholin's cyst. It can be really painful and at the very least will need antibiotic treatment and at the worst surgery. So if you notice a small swelling near the opening of your vagina, go straight to your doctor before it gets worse.

The Vagina

The word vagina derives from the Latin word for sheath or scabbard. It varies in size from woman to woman but is about 8cm long.

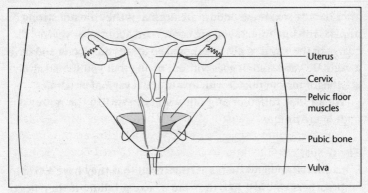

Uterus

Cervix

Pelvic floor muscles

Pubic bone

Vulva

Vagina

When it's not in use it is closed and its two sides touch each other. Your vagina has your vulva at the outer end and your cervix and uterus at the inner end. Your vagina is a very elastic and muscular organ that can stretch when aroused to allow the entry of a penis; after you have had sex your vagina quickly returns to its normal closed state. It is a myth to think that once you have lost your virginity your vagina is permanently stretched. Your vagina also stretches considerably to allow the birth of a baby. If you are young your vagina will return more or less to how it was before with some pelvic floor rehabilitation. However, as we are all having babies later it's worth saying if you are having children over the age of thirty-five you need to take more care of your pelvic floor afterwards as your vagina ages just like the rest of your body. Your vagina is sometimes called the birth canal in books about pregnancy and childbirth. It is also the place where blood flows down during your menstrual cycle.

Your vagina is self-cleaning, meaning that you do not need to use douches, creams or gels up there and it is much healthier to avoid scented products or strong soaps. Vaginal discharge is usually perfectly normal and this changes throughout your menstrual cycle; some women can tell when they are fertile by the amount of vaginal secretion or mucus, while others have much less secretion. Vaginal smells vary throughout your cycle and sometimes after having sex; these odours are normal if they are not strong or unpleasant-smelling. If you are concerned about your vaginal discharge or the way it smells you should go to see your doctor and have a vaginal swab taken. It goes without saying that you should always go straight to your doctor with any unusual vaginal bleeding.

We all look different and our vaginas, just like the rest of our bodies, are unique.

The G Spot

Is it a myth? Some women are convinced that they have a G spot while others can feel like they are a sexual failure if they never have an orgasm with vaginal penetration. There is absolutely no point spending your life worrying that you are not normal. We are all different – and thank goodness! It matters not how sexual arousal occurs as long as you are enjoying it. Despite lots of research it remains unproven as to whether the G spot exists and, if it does, where it is. So please don't add this to your list of things to worry about.

Vaginal Wind

As with many other things we've covered in this book, vaginal wind is consistently under-reported. When it happens it often sounds like normal flatulence, and can sometimes feel like bubbles being released. If it's happening to you in the middle of a passionate sexual experience at best it may cause a fit of the giggles or at worst it could put you off sex for ever.

This can occur after having children due to weak and lax pelvic floor muscles. It can also occur when you have not had any children and the action of your partner's penis going in and out can cause air to become trapped in your vagina. It can happen with the insertion of fingers, sex aids or toys. It can also happen when you are having a smear test or any type of vaginal examination when a vaginal speculum is inserted, drawing air in with it.

It can also happen in the middle of a very quiet yoga class, which can be highly embarrassing. It sometimes occurs when you do a headstand as air is sucked into the weak vagina and released as you move. If this is happening to you please do something about it; it's not something you just have to put up with. You need to take action if you are nodding while reading this bit.

The difference between vaginal wind and normal farting is that with vaginal wind you have no control over it whatsoever.

Urinary Incontinence During Sex

This can be a very distressing thing to experience. Incontinence can happen during sex or at the point of orgasm but is often mistaken for extra lubrication caused by sexual arousal.

This is yet another under-reported problem. In my experience women rarely come to see me because they are having urinary incontinence during sex. That doesn't mean that I have never come across anyone with the problem – far from it. There is a high prevalence of incontinence during sex in women who have urinary incontinence in their normal life. This is usually stress incontinence (see Chapter 3) but an overactive bladder (see Chapter 4) may also cause leaking at orgasm.

This is something that women only tell me about if I ask them directly. Then they will often say, 'Oh yes, it's been happening since I had the children. I always put a towel on the bed, just in case.' It can be very embarrassing, affect your ability to have an orgasm and even cause problems with your relationship.

In general, this problem occurs as a result of weak pelvic floor muscles, so this is your moment to start strengthening your muscles (see Chapter 2). It is also helpful to try to double void before sex (see page 23). Avoid drinks high in caffeine prior to sex and try sex positions that put less pressure on your bladder. Last but not least, talk to your partner about it, as most men will completely understand.

Vaginal Laxity

Vaginal laxity is when you have little or no sensation during intercourse. Vaginal laxity may also exist if you have stress incontinence. Vaginal laxity often occurs after having children and is more likely to happen if you have had more than one child, if your baby was very large at birth or if you had an assisted delivery, perhaps with forceps. I do see vaginal laxity in young women who have not yet had a baby, although these women have usually come to see me with chronic constipation (see Chapter 9) and are sometimes hypermobile (see page 66).

Vaginal laxity may seem to be a small problem to have but it can really affect your quality of life so it's really important to seek treatment.

I remember treating a lady a while ago who came to see me as she had stress incontinence. She had three teenage boys all of whom had been vaginal deliveries and all huge babies. When I first examined her I asked her to contract her pelvic floor muscles and nothing happened at all. I then connected her to my biofeedback machine (I use a vaginal probe that you squeeze with your vaginal muscles) and I asked her to contract her muscles again. This time she could see on my computer screen that barely anything was happening at all. She was horrified and determined to do something about it. At this point she had told me that her sex life was fine, apart from the fact that she and her husband didn't do it as often as they used to as they were both so busy working and caring for the family. I decided to treat her with electrical stimulation; there was little point in her trying to do pelvic floor exercises as she had such a limited ability to contract her muscles. After a few months we were chatting and looking at her much improved muscle tone on my computer when she blurted out, 'I had sex with my husband the other day and I can honestly tell you that I had totally forgotten what it used to feel like. It's amazing! After having the boys my vagina just got looser and looser and all sensation had disappeared. I now have my vagina and my sex life back and my stress incontinence is cured.'

Orgasms

An orgasm is a feeling of intense sexual pleasure that happens during sexual activity, which results in rhythmic contractions in the pelvic region. Orgasms can be achieved in different ways; the most normal way is with clitoral stimulation either with a partner or with masturbation. It can also happen with vaginal or anal penetration or oral sex. For some people (amazingly) it can happen in their dreams. You have possibly chatted to your girlfriends about your orgasms – it's generally a lot easier than talking about stress incontinence.

For some women orgasms seem to come easily and they are able to have lots of them. Others find them hard to achieve and regularly do a bit of faking. Whatever is happening to you, as long as you are enjoying your orgasms embrace them and be happy. If you are not achieving orgasms or they are not as you think they should be, please do something about it. We know that when women regularly perform their pelvic floor exercises this can have positive effects on female sexual function.[26] This is good news for us all!

Vulvodynia

Vulvodynia is chronic vulval pain that feels like burning or stinging. It can be constant or intermittent. The British Association of Dermatologists says that vulvodynia affects 15 per cent of women. It can make sitting down painful; riding a bike can also be very unpleasant. It may hurt just wearing your skinny jeans. It can be triggered by touch with sexual intercourse or when trying to insert a tampon. If really severe it can make sexual intercourse impossible.

Sadly it can be a difficult condition to diagnose, as there are no visible symptoms and no known cause of the pain. Try to think of it a bit like migraine – it's a type of complex regional pain syndrome. There is no simple cure but there is a lot of help out there so please don't suffer in silence.[27] The British Society for the Study of Vulval Diseases has a map of vulval clinics and services in the

UK where you can get the help that you need (see Helpful Organizations, page 158).

While you are waiting for your appointment it might help to:

- Perform your pelvic floor exercises but please stop if it makes things worse.
- Wear cotton underwear.
- Sit on a cushion with a hole in the middle.
- Apply a cool pack to your vulva.
- Use a local anaesthetic gel ten minutes before you have intercourse.
- During sex try different positions to see which ones work the best.
- Your doctor may prescribe medication to help you, or may suggest using TENS (transcutaneous electrical nerve stimulation).

Dyspareunia (Painful Sex)

According to the Sexual Advice Association painful sex is thought to affect between 8 and 22 per cent of women. This is a shocking statistic. When I ask my patients whether they are sexually active they often reveal that they are not, even when they are in a long-term relationship. It's amazing how many people are not sexually active because of pain, loss of self-image or fear following childbirth. A 2017 study that was published in the *British Journal of Obstetrics and Gynaecology: An International Journal of Obstetrics and Gynaecology* found that nearly one in ten British women experience painful sex. Interestingly (and I suppose not hugely surprisingly) the two largest groups reporting painful sex were the group aged sixteen to twenty-four and the group aged fifty-five to sixty-four. It was also reported that painful sex was strongly associated with vaginal dryness, feeling anxious during sex and lack of sexual enjoyment.

While painful sex is a common problem it's often overlooked, as it's an extremely intimate problem. If you are experiencing painful sex (or have given up having sex due to pain) then it may help to use lubricating gels or oils – there are lots of good ones on the market like Yes or Sylk and you can buy them online if you feel shy about buying them in the pharmacy.

If you are postnatal or menopausal then vaginal oestrogen may be the answer. Vaginal dilators can help and at the same time build confidence (see page 96). It's always a good idea to lose weight if necessary and avoid getting constipated (see Chapter 9) as that can make sex uncomfortable or even painful. There is evidence that practising pelvic floor exercises probably helps dyspareunia.[28] It may also be worthwhile considering counselling or sexual therapy, and sometimes cognitive behavioural therapy can help if everything to do with sex has become negative.

Lichen Planus and Lichen Sclerosus

You may not know that you have either of these conditions – they are both conditions that can affect the skin of the vulva. You may be just having really painful sexual intercourse or have stopped being able to have penetrative sex. By reading this and having a look at your vulva, hopefully some of you at the early stages of these problems can get help and treatment sooner.

The symptoms of both these conditions can be itchy, sore or fragile skin around your vulva and around the anus as well. Quite often your vulval skin will have changed colour. It does tend to affect older women, so with the menopause and possible atrophic vaginitis (see page 88) on top, sex may well have become a distant memory. Use a mirror to check whether your vulval skin has changed colour or looks different; if your skin looks pale, whitish or reddish-brown and blotchy please go to see your doctor. There is sadly no cure for these two problems but the symptoms can certainly be relieved or reduced, usually with creams and sometimes with tablets, so do seek help. You may need to have more tests or a biopsy to find out if it is either lichen planus or lichen sclerosus. If it proves to be one of these two conditions don't worry; they are not contagious so you can't give it to your partner. They are both chronic conditions that affect the skin of the vulva, the cause of which is not really understood as yet.

Vaginismus

I am covering vaginismus separately from dyspareunia but they do partially overlap in terms of symptoms. I hope that keeping them separate will help you to work out exactly which one you have and how it is best treated. If treated correctly there is a good chance that you will recover and go on to have a normal sex life.

Vaginismus happens as a result of an involuntary contraction of the vaginal/pelvic floor muscles. It is when the muscles of your vagina tighten so that they either limit or prevent penetration. Women often say it feels like something is 'hitting a wall'. If penetration does happen it can be extremely painful and distressing. There is then naturally a fear of having sex even when you really want to. It can happen while trying to have sex, inserting a tampon or possibly having a smear test. It is not something that you have control over. It may occur even if you have been using tampons and having sex normally in the past, but it is far more common among young girls or women when they first try to use a tampon or have sex. At the moment doctors don't really know what causes vaginismus but possible reasons could be fear that penetration will be painful; recurrent painful medical conditions like thrush or urinary tract infections; a bad first sexual encounter; or maybe you feel that sex is somehow shameful or wrong.

As you can imagine, if you have this particular problem vaginal examination is very stressful so it is very difficult to conduct research into this problem.

To treat vaginismus you can start by looking at your vulva and vagina in a mirror just to get used to what you look like. It will hopefully take away some of the mystery of how you look down there. You can then start a programme of pelvic floor exercises (see Chapter 2). This will help give you more control over your vaginal muscles. Once you have been doing this for a week or two then you can start trying to insert either your finger or a small vaginal dilator with some lubricant or local anaesthetic gel into your vagina (you should discuss this first with your doctor or healthcare practitioner). You may find doing this (particularly if you are using your finger) easiest in the bath.

Whatever you do don't feel shy or embarrassed about seeking help. You may need the help of a specialist, whether a gynaecologist, a pelvic floor specialist or a psychosexual counsellor (see Helpful Organizations, page 158). You may also find that the practice of sensate focus (see page 116) is of benefit.

Men and Sex

With men it's difficult to ignore your genitals as unlike women's they are not neatly tucked away. For men sex and sexual arousal involves an erection, which can happen with physical or psychological stimulation or both. But sometimes things are not working quite how they should and I hope that this next bit of my book will help you to sort out your worries and hopefully face them. Even if the only reason that you are reading this section is because your partner bought my book and came upon this bit and thought to herself, 'this is us', do please read it. I hope that what it says will benefit you both.

Premature Ejaculation

A recent study suggests that premature ejaculation (PE) subjectively affects 20–30 per cent of men globally.[29] It means that when you ejaculate (come) it all happens too soon, but it is important to note, as the study does, that this is a very subjective experience. Many couples are extremely happy with their sex lives so I do not want to create a problem where there isn't one. However, if coming too soon is bothering you then I hope that the information below will help you.

An average man will have an ejaculation between 4 and 8 minutes after vaginal penetration. In contrast, premature ejaculation occurs about one minute after penetration and sometimes even before penetration.

The reason for PE may be multi-faceted. It could be that it happened during your first sexual experience and your partner wasn't very understanding or was unkind and so you have an anxiety about sexual performance. It could be stress-related or it may also be a medical problem. If PE is caused by a medical problem, please seek help from your doctor straight away. It may have started when you were young, either when you were trying to masturbate quickly in case anyone caught you, or were having sex at your girlfriend's house and were terrified that her parents might come home. There are many reasons why PE happens and there are also lots of self-help solutions.

If you are suffering from PE please do not think that you are alone – think of the other 20–30 per cent of the population who have the same troubles as you.

There is good evidence to suggest that pelvic floor exercises (see Chapter 2) can play a part in helping you to improve premature ejaculation. They are so easy to do, can be done anywhere and require hardly any time at all. So get started today!

You can use a couple of different techniques to try to build tolerance to delay ejaculation. One is called pause–squeeze and the other is called stop–start. In the pause–squeeze techniques, you masturbate yourself (or of course your partner can help you) almost to the point of orgasm and then stop and hold the end of your penis tightly. Repeat the process four or five times. The next time allow ejaculation to occur.

The other way is stop–start: this is where you masturbate to the point of ejaculation then stop and wait until your arousal level is diminished. Repeat the process about three times and then on the next go allow ejaculation to occur.

You can practise either of these techniques as often as you wish. After practising for a few weeks the feeling of knowing how to delay ejaculation might become more normal and hopefully you will have learned to control your ejaculations and allow them to happen a little later. Masturbating an hour or two before having sex also helps some people.

There are drugs available to help, in particular a drug called Dapoxetine (Priligy). This is the first drug to be licensed in the UK to treat premature ejaculation. You will need to get this from your doctor on prescription.

Sometimes it is recommended that you apply a numbing or anaesthetic cream to your penis a few minutes before intercourse. However, if you do this you will also need to wear a condom or you may cause numbness to your partner's vagina.

If you have tried some of the options above and are still having issues you may want to consider sexual therapy.

Erectile Dysfunction

Erectile dysfunction (ED) or impotence is a common problem and about half of men between forty and seventy have it to a degree. If you are unsure whether or not you are suffering from this problem then take a look at the Helpful Organizations on pages 158 ('Sex') and 159 ('Men') for links to organizations that can help. You could also visit your doctor who may refer you to a urologist: many of them will use the questionnaire over the page, which you might find useful.[30] This can help both you and your doctor assess the issue to manage your erectile dysfunction effectively.

Most men at some point in their lives will fail to get an erection or lose it halfway through the act of making love. This is totally normal and nothing to worry about. It can be caused by stress, tiredness or excessive alcohol consumption. It might be that your relationship is in injury time and the spark has gone out. This doesn't mean there is anything wrong with you. You need to remember this, as ED can start happening due to fear of failure. Or you may never get to the fear of failure point as you have just given up even trying. Erectile dysfunction only becomes a cause for concern with action required if the problem keeps happening.

There are physical reasons sometimes why erectile dysfunction starts to happen so I do urge you to have a general health check if it has started happening to you out of the blue. Some of the things

If you are not sure that you have erectile dysfunction, here is a quick and easy guide to help you.

Sexual Health Inventory for Men (SHIM)

Instructions

Each question has five possible responses. Circle the number that best describes your own situation. Select only one answer for each question.

Over the last six months:

1. How do you rate your confidence that you could keep an erection?

1	2	3	4	5
Very low	Low	Moderate	High	Very high

2. When you had erections with sexual stimulation, how often were your erections hard enough for penetration (entering your partner)?

1	2	3	4	5
Almost never or never	A few times (much less than half the time)	Sometimes (about half the time)	Most times (more than half the time)	Almost always or always

3. During sexual intercourse, how often were you able to maintain your erection after you had penetrated (entered) your partner?

1	2	3	4	5
Almost never or never	A few times (much less than half the time)	Sometimes (about half the time)	Most times (more than half the time)	Almost always or always

4. During sexual intercourse, how difficult was it to maintain your erection to completion of intercourse?

1	2	3	4	5
Extremely difficult	Very difficult	Difficult	Slightly difficult	Not difficult

5. When you attempted sexual intercourse, how often was it satisfactory for you?

1	2	3	4	5
Almost never or never	A few times (much less than half the time)	Sometimes (about half the time)	Most times (more than half the time)	Almost always or always

that can bring it on are heart disease, high blood pressure, high cholesterol, diabetes or following a radical prostatectomy (see page 143). Please don't be alarmed, but do go and have a check-up.

Every week I ask women if they are sexually active and far too often they tell me, 'I would love to be but my husband is finding it hard to keep his erections, so we have given up that part of our lives.' This is a huge shame. Often my patients say their partners are very reluctant to discuss it with a doctor. It's a taboo subject just like urinary incontinence but we must do something to change this. If this is you and you recognize yourself go and find help at once.

Here are some self-help techniques:

- Try to lose weight if you are overweight.
- Give up smoking.
- Try to improve your lifestyle by eating a more healthy diet, reducing your alcohol intake and doing some exercise. In the process you may have the added benefits of lowering your cholesterol and your blood pressure – all good news for your future.
- Try to reduce your stress levels.
- Start doing pelvic floor exercises. We know that your pelvic floor muscles are active during sexual intercourse and play a role in penile erection (see Chapter 2).

- Try not to cycle for more than three hours a week and if you do, make sure that you have a very cushioned or padded seat. It's possible you are squashing the blood vessels and nerves supplying your penis. There's no point being super-fit but suffering ED as a result.

If the lifestyle changes have not worked or not completely worked the next step would be medication, so you will need to discuss this with your doctor. However, if you can't take the medication or you don't wish to then it's a good idea to find a sexual therapist who can guide you through the alternative treatments that are available. They can include:

- A pellet that you put down the end of your penis – when it dissolves it gives you an erection
- The use of a pump or vacuum device. The vacuum draws blood into your penis and causes an erection
- Injections into your penis
- Penile implants

It may be that you need sex therapy and this could be on your own or as part of couples counselling. Sex therapy is considered highly effective in addressing the main causes of sexual difficulties. Do check out the website of the Sexual Advice Association (see Helpful Organizations, page 158).

Sensate Focus
Finally, I wanted to highlight a technique called sensate focus that can be used if you or your partner is experiencing any kind of sexual problem. It was developed by Masters and Johnson in the 1960s and is widely used by sexual health therapists. The technique involves touching and stroking and being touched and stroked. Through mindful caressing of each other's body you get to know your partner's body and what they really like, where they like to be touched and what makes them happy. Sensate focus

begins with non-genital touching. Slowly you get to know and enjoy each other's body. As you get to know each other's body better you then move on to touching first breasts and then your genital area until you are able to give each other an orgasm. You can then move on to sexual intercourse. This process is best done in conjunction with a trained sexual therapist.

NINE

Your Bowels

Bowels are not glamorous. Going for a poo is something we all do in private so we don't talk about it to each other, even when things aren't going as they should.

The pelvic floor is very important to help you poo properly and there are various muscles and nerves involved in the process illustrated below.

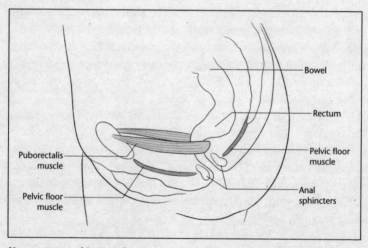

Your rectum and its muscles

The puborectalis muscle hooks round your rectum in a sling-like way. It works either to keep you continent (so you don't poo yourself) or to relax in conjunction with your anal sphincter so that you can open your bowels. Problems happen when these muscles and/or the nerves around them are damaged in some way.

Bowel dysfunction can have many causes; here are some of the main ones:

- Chronic constipation and straining on the toilet
- Childbirth damaging the muscles or nerves you use to control your bowels
- Long-term irritable bowel syndrome (IBS)
- Pelvic floor disorders
- Other reasons why your bowels may suddenly misbehave include having an operation, illness, pregnancy, periods of anxiety in your life, long-term misuse of laxatives, new medication, haemorrhoids or anal fissures (tearing in the anus)

The gastrointestinal or digestive tract is long; it starts at the point where we eat food and ends at the anus when we expel our faeces or poo. It takes approximately 1–3 days for the whole process to work. We take in food at one end, extract the nutrients and things we need from it and then expel the rest as waste. This is, of course, in an ideal world when your bowels are working like a well-oiled machine.

I am sure that all of us at some point in our lives have had a 'bowel issue'. It's always unpleasant, whether it's constipation, diarrhoea, bloating, pain, nausea, vomiting or wind – at the least it can be inconvenient and at worst it's downright distressing. Most of us simply rush to the chemist, buy something to make us either go or stop going and are relieved when equilibrium is restored.

Constipation

Constipation can both be the cause of and be caused by pelvic floor dysfunction. It is not a visible thing: you are not wetting yourself nor are you running to the toilet all day. Nevertheless if you are suffering from constipation, it can be as life-changing as any of the other issues discussed in this book. It can become all-consuming, taking over your life. Constipation can be caused by lots of things:

- Not being active enough
- Not drinking enough water
- Consuming too little fibre in your diet
- Medication
- Vaginal prolapse (see Chapter 5)
- Resisting the urge to poo (this can sometimes start in childhood)
- Haemorrhoids or anal fissures (which can make you scared to poo due to the pain)
- Pregnancy and the initial couple of months following childbirth
- Slow transit of faeces within your colon
- Pelvic floor dysfunction
- Irritable bowel syndrome
- Certain medical conditions

Constipation can also be a symptom of colon cancer so if you have any concerns you should go straight to your GP.

Here is a classic example of when things have all gone wrong. Quite often I ask my patients when their constipation started and the answer is often when they were a child. Sometimes being asked, 'Have you been?' and knowing if you said no some horrid-tasting medicine or a trip to the doctor would follow, the answer was always, 'Yes, I went this morning.'

A common fear is not wanting to open your bowels in public places. What if there are noises or, heaven forbid, smells? Is there any toilet paper? Possibly it's not wanting to sit on a toilet seat that isn't your own; hovering over the toilet is not an ideal position for effective bowel movements. I am sure we have all done this on at least one occasion. I bet you have thought to yourself, goodness, there are people I know in the toilets so I'm too embarrassed to poo here. Most of the time we can put off the urge to defecate until we are in a place we prefer, preferably at home with the door locked. But we shouldn't feel so embarrassed about opening our bowels, it is something we all do on a regular basis, yet even today we still remain very coy about the whole process.

One good example of this is a woman who came to see me with a rectocele (a prolapse of the back wall of the vagina, see Chapter 5). She came for pelvic floor rehabilitation but when I examined her I realized that she was very constipated. It turned out that she always needed to poo in the morning right at the same time as the school run so she was consistently not able to go when she needed to. After dropping off the children the urge often had passed and an awful cycle had begun. Eventually this led to her prolapse. I am sure this is familiar to some of you reading this. Even when our pace of life is totally frenetic we need to take a step back and care for our basic bodily functions or face worse problems in the future. This woman described having to put her fingers in her vagina to push the prolapse back into place in order to empty her bowels. This sounds shocking, but something similar is going on a lot behind closed doors. So don't feel alone with this problem – start doing something about it.

Another woman with young children told me that she absolutely needed to smoke a cigarette and drink a coffee in order to poo. This was proving ever more difficult as her young children were getting older and wiser. She had 'given up' smoking years before and was truly terrified that the children or her husband might catch her at it! Come rain, hail or shine she could be found at the bottom of the garden behind the shed, having her illicit cigarette – all to be able to poo!

Dyssynergic Defecation

Dyssynergic defecation is an inability to coordinate your abdominal and pelvic floor muscles to poo. It is an under-diagnosed problem with many people never having heard of it. It affects about 50 per cent of people with chronic constipation. How many of us go to the doctor and say, I don't think I am pooing properly? We are soon there if there is pain or blood in our poo but a bit of straining? I don't think so.

Dyssynergic defecation is a type of pelvic floor dysfunction and is quite often present without urinary problems, although some patients do come to see me with this problem and on questioning them they will admit to a bit of stress incontinence. Once again, it's not normal, even after having children, but it reveals the massive amount of under-reported or under-diagnosed urinary and bladder problems in the population. With the right treatment (biofeedback therapy and possibly laxatives) you can get a lot better. You may possibly need some tests (either an X-ray or MRI scan, or you may have a balloon put in your bottom to see if you are able to push it out – a balloon expulsion test) by your doctor, gastroenterologist or pelvic floor specialist to find an accurate diagnosis.

Symptoms of constipation are:

- Straining to poo
- Going to the toilet less than three times per week
- Passing hard, dry and lumpy stools
- Having a lot of bloating or stomach cramps
- Having to put your fingers either into your vagina or rectum to empty yourself
- Often feeling that you haven't emptied your bowels properly

Treating Constipation

To help sort out your constipation you will probably need to do a variety of things. The way we sit on the toilet may be more important than we think. Lots of people tell me they put their feet up on their children's toilet step, the bathroom bin or even a couple of toilet rolls. Sometimes they just pull their knees up to their chin. I am sure that we have all wriggled about on the toilet in order 'to go', maybe when we are in a hurry or a bit constipated.

All you need is something that elevates your knees above your hips so that you are in a natural squatting position. The reason for this is that our bowels have a natural bend (the anorectal angle),

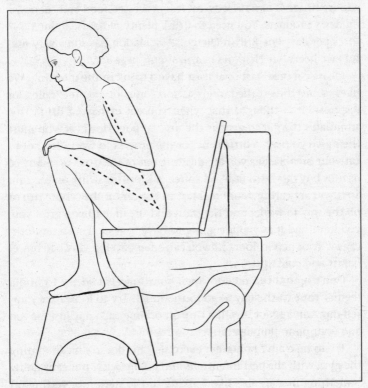

Using a footstool to help open your bowels

which is important in keeping us continent; your puborectalis muscle helps to maintain this angle. So when you poo your puborectalis muscle needs to relax so that you can go effectively. Often the act of bearing down causes the muscle to relax, straightening out the rectum. However, the squatting position possibly helps to relax your puborectalis muscle a little more to help you to go.

This is certainly not necessary for all of us but nearly all of my patients with constipation have found using a raised footstool helpful.

Make sure that you have enough high-fibre foods including vegetables, fruits, cereals and wholegrain foods in your diet. Try adding linseeds or flaxseeds, eat less processed food and cut down on dairy products. You need to drink plenty of fluids, about 1.5–2 litres per day. The British Dietetic Association has some very useful factsheets (see Helpful Organizations, page 155)

Please eat breakfast or at least have a drink in the morning. We have something called the gastrocolonic or colonic reflex or response; it is thought that when you eat or have a drink this stimulates the gut to give us the urge to poo. However, you must then give yourself a little time for the process to work. Try not to eat your breakfast as you are dashing out of the door. So many of us now buy our breakfast and coffee or morning drink on the run. So if you are eating your breakfast in the car on the school run or on the way to work or on the train and the urge to poo grips you, you have had it as you are going to have to wait. This does nothing for your pelvic floor and you can then develop very bad bowel habits and constipation.

Don't ignore the urge to open your bowels and try to find a regular time in the day to go to the toilet. Try to look after yourself more and give yourself a tiny bit of time each day just for you and your poor old bowels!

Try to take a bit of regular exercise. This doesn't mean joining the gym with the best intentions and going twice. It means doing something manageable like walking to the station or getting off the bus a stop earlier than usual. Always use the stairs – a good tip is to walk up the escalators or get out of the lift a few floors before your one. It's these baby steps that will lead to a healthier lifestyle and better bowel habits.

It's possible that you may need to take laxatives and a visit to your pharmacist or doctor will be required to find the appropriate medication. There is nothing wrong with this so don't feel embarrassed. It's much more important to sort out your constipation than doing further damage to your pelvic floor muscles and ending up with a prolapse or haemorrhoids.

The chart below was created to help all healthcare professionals

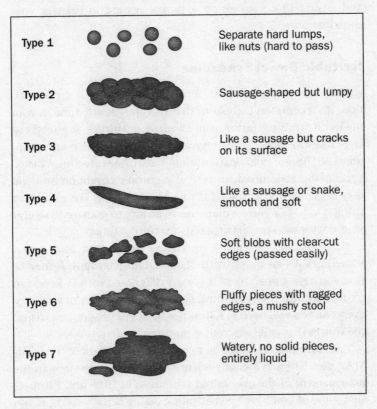

Type 1		Separate hard lumps, like nuts (hard to pass)
Type 2		Sausage-shaped but lumpy
Type 3		Like a sausage but cracks on its surface
Type 4		Like a sausage or snake, smooth and soft
Type 5		Soft blobs with clear-cut edges (passed easily)
Type 6		Fluffy pieces with ragged edges, a mushy stool
Type 7		Watery, no solid pieces, entirely liquid

The Bristol stool chart

explain to everyone what your poo is meant to look like. It's a brilliant tool and if you are not sure if your poo looks like good healthy poo (as stool types 3 and 4), have a look at the chart on the previous page. It shows in detail what you can't really ask anyone and may make you realize that something is not right.

I have seen lots of people who know that when they are constipated it's harder to empty their bladder. Sometimes there are other issues: for example in men, an enlarged prostate; in women, fibroids or prolapse may be an added problem. Severe constipation can also lead to faecal incontinence so you must seek help and ensure that you are on a proper regime to manage your constipation.

Irritable Bowel Syndrome

Irritable bowel syndrome affects about 10 per cent of the population. It's a common complaint that can start at any time in your life but it tends to start in your twenties or thirties. It affects the large intestine and can vary greatly in severity. The main symptoms of IBS are constipation and/or diarrhoea, feeling bloated and having abdominal pains. It is a chronic condition and you may suffer with it on and off throughout your life. The important thing is to have a correct diagnosis to be able to manage it, so visit your doctor who can arrange tests for the condition.

It is possible that you have lactose or fructose intolerance. Sometimes it's an overgrowth of bacteria in your gut. It may be that you have a slow colon. If you are diagnosed with IBS you can try to deal with the symptoms, but as no one treatment works for everyone you will need to follow the advice of your doctor to find the things that will help your symptoms.

I am sure that some of you have heard or read about the FOD-MAP diet. There is lots of evidence about its effectiveness in the management of the abdominal symptoms of IBS[31] and I suspect that some of you have been avoiding eating certain foods as you know that they make your symptoms worse. FODMAP stands for fermentable, oligosaccharides, disaccharides, monosaccharides and polyols. These are a group of simple and complex sugars that are not very well absorbed by the body and are found in vegetables, fruit, milk and wheat. If you wish to try the FODMAP diet you should ask to be referred to a dietitian, as it's very important you are eating food that will give you the right nutritional content.

Irritable bowel syndrome can lead to pelvic floor dysfunction. This is mainly due to constipation but lots of repeated diarrhoea can also cause pelvic floor weakness. As this is a condition that tends to start when you are relatively young and can go on for many years, please don't forget your pelvic floor exercises along the way.

Haemorrhoids

Haemorrhoids (also known as piles) are swollen, enlarged and inflamed veins either in your rectum or around your anus. They may happen when you are pregnant and especially in the third trimester, but hopefully after delivery of your baby the symptoms will resolve themselves. They may have no discernible cause but being overweight is a factor, as is age – as we get older all our tissues become weaker, even the ones around your bottom. Spending a long time reading the newspaper on the toilet is also to be avoided as this allows the veins of your anus to fill with blood so they are under more pressure. And, of course, straining to poo is also a factor.

Piles can be internal so you may not know you have them unless they bleed or are painful; as always if you see any blood from your bottom you must see your doctor, however embarrassing it may be. External haemorrhoids are more visible and may itch or be painful.

If they are not bad enough to send you running to your doctor, look after yourself by following the advice on treating constipation (see page 123). The next step is to try over-the-counter creams or suppositories but if these don't work your doctor can prescribe stronger medication for you.

There is a surgical solution in the form of rubber band ligation. This is simply a tight band that is put around your haemorrhoid to cut off the blood supply; the haemorrhoid will dry up and fall off. If your condition is very severe then you may need to have a haemorrhoidectomy. This is an operation to remove them and is definitely a last resort after you have tried everything else.

A friend of mine told me that every time she moved house (and this was a lot as her husband was in the army) she had terrible constipation and this inevitably led to haemorrhoids or piles. So off to a new doctor she would go and show him her bottom. Inevitably a few weeks later he would be sitting at her dinner table making polite conversation. She tells me that after this has happened a few times you simply have to get over your blushes and get on with it. So I hope her open and honest story helps some of you to feel the same.

Anal Fissures

Anal fissures are a small tear or little ulcer at the entrance of your anus. They may cause bleeding in the form of bright red blood when you wipe your bottom. If you have this problem then it will undoubtedly make you want to not poo as the pain may be eye-watering. They usually heal in a few weeks but they can be chronic. To treat anal fissures follow the treatment for constipation (see page 123).

Sometimes creams can help but always seek your doctor's advice to ensure you have the right treatment. As with haemorrhoids, a surgical solution for your anal fissure is always the last resort.

Uncontrolled Wind

We all pass wind regularly throughout the day, on average anywhere between five and fifteen times a day. In general, we do it silently or when no one else is listening. But when it starts happening and we simply have no control over it please don't think it's the end of the world. It can be helped or even cured, usually with a mixture of dietary changes, good bowel habits and pelvic floor rehabilitation. If it's appropriate I sometimes use electrical stimulation of the pelvic floor to treat uncontrolled wind as it helps to improve muscle tone in very weak pelvic floor muscles and possible postnatal nerve damage.

I have looked after many women who are struggling to control wind. This is highly embarrassing in public but can be equally dreadful in front of family members. A wonderful patient of mine told me that when it happens to her it is usually because she has eaten sprouts or a few other foods that cause the problem. But she also told me that after doing her pelvic floor exercises for a week or two things are always much better. Another patient told me about a recent incident with her grandson, who had asked her to read him a story. As she bent down to get the book she could not control her wind and let out a loud noise. Her wide-eyed grandson simply said, 'Oh, Mrs Fart.' She was able to smile as she told me the story and was desperate to sort out her pelvic floor so it never happened again.

Faecal Urgency and Incontinence

Faecal urgency is an urgent desire to open your bowels, whereas faecal incontinence is actual loss of bowel control. If you think this is not very common, statistics show that about 10 per cent of women suffer from one of the above or uncontrolled wind after childbirth.

Faecal incontinence really is life-changing. It can occur following childbirth particularly if you have had a third- or fourth-degree tear (obstetric anal sphincter injury). It involves damage to your anal sphincter and, in a fourth-degree tear, the tear gets bigger and damages the lining of your anus and possibly the rectum itself. This is more likely to happen in new mothers over the age of thirty-five, with large babies and in a forceps or ventouse delivery.

If any of you are reading this and have faecal leakage, faecal urgency or faecal incontinence please seek help (see Helpful Organizations, page 157). The MASIC Foundation (Mothers with Anal Sphincter Injuries in Childbirth) is there for you as a starting point if you are struggling to tell anyone what is happening to you. Whatever you do, don't suffer in silence.

There are a variety of things you can do to improve the situation. Pelvic floor exercises are a must and I would recommend electrical stimulation of the muscles to start with. If the nerves that keep you continent are damaged beyond repair, then a management strategy is required. This can be tough stuff, particularly with a new baby.

Easy access to toilets is vital while out and about. You are allowed to use disabled toilets and it may help to obtain a card from your local continence nurse specialist, called the 'Just Can't Wait' toilet card (see Helpful Organizations, page 160). There is also a national key scheme called RADAR, which allows you access to about 8,000 public toilets around the country. You can get the key from the local council, some healthcare professionals or buy one online.

Certain foods can make things worse. If you already have a healthy diet then it's a good idea to keep a food diary for at least a week so you can see if anything makes the problems worse.

Treatments for Faecal Urgency and Incontinence
Anal Plug
You can wear an anal plug for security and there are a few on the market (Renew inserts and Peristeen anal plug to name but two). Some of these are available to buy over the counter and some are available only on prescription.

Loperamide (Imodium)
This is a drug that is available on prescription and over the counter. It can be helpful in controlling faecal urgency or faecal

incontinence and can be used as required, for example if you are worried that you may have an accident when you are going to an important engagement. It is used to treat diarrhoea and can slow down your bowel and make your poo a little less loose. However, you should not use this in certain circumstances – for example, if you are pregnant – so please read the instructions carefully and check with your doctor or pharmacist before taking any medication.

Peristeen irrigation

This and other forms of trans anal irrigation can be very useful. Some of them are available only on prescription from your doctor and all of them must be taught correctly by a properly trained healthcare professional. They work by emptying your rectum with water irrigation. You do this by inserting a small catheter into your anus while you are sitting on the toilet. When you instil the water your bowel is stimulated to empty. It is something that you can do every day or every other day, depending on the exact problem you're experiencing. If you are having severe constipation or faecal incontinence this may improve your quality of life a lot, as you are able to use it at a time to suit you, giving you the freedom to go about your daily life with less worry of feeling uncomfortable or having an accident. I had a patient who was working in a very busy office and she was terrified of having an accident at work. By irrigating her rectum before leaving the house she was able to manage her problem and carry on with the job she loved.

Neuromodulation (Sacral Nerve Stimulation)

This involves placing a small electronic device under your skin, usually at the top of one buttock. It can help the muscles and nerves in your anus to work better. It is something that may be tried if conservative measures have failed. It is a minimally invasive treatment but has to be performed in a hospital or specialist clinic and could help to restore your continence.

Tibial Nerve Stimulation
This can be helpful if you have faecal urgency or faecal incontinence (see Chapter 4).

Surgery
Surgery for faecal incontinence is always the last resort. It involves an operation to repair the damaged muscles in your anus; the most commonly performed procedure is a sphincteroplasty.

TEN

Everyone Has a Pelvic Floor: Advice for Men

The male pelvic floor is a hammock of muscle stretching from your tailbone at the back to the pubic bone at the front, and between the bones that you sit on, from one side to the other. It is a very important structure and one that you probably have never even given a second thought to if it has been working well for you. Your urethra and your anus both pass through your pelvic floor and your pelvic floor works to keep you continent both of urine and faeces, stop you passing wind at inappropriate times and plays an important part in getting and maintaining erections and in having orgasms.

The male pelvic floor has been discussed throughout history and was first mentioned in Egyptian manuscripts in 1500 BC, where papyrus leaves were used 'to remove constant running of urine'.[32] In the seventeenth century urinals were being fashioned out of pigs' bladders to be worn over the penis and catch any urine loss. It was also at this time that the first penile clamps to prevent leakage were invented. All this must have been a great improvement on wet clothing, particularly in a time when there were no washing machines or tumble dryers.

In the early twentieth century we had moved on to urinals made of India rubber. We are still using this method today in the

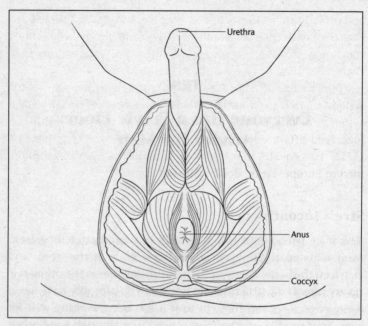

Male pelvic floor

form of a penile sheath and leg bag, although of course they are now made from medical-grade silicone and are much more reliable, comfortable and easy to use. In 1929 a man called Frederick Foley pioneered the first self-retaining balloon catheter. If any of you have had an operation and woken up with a catheter in your penis this is still called a Foley catheter nearly one hundred years later. For our purposes it would only be used as a very last resort for intractable urinary incontinence but it is a wonderful invention and in design is largely unchanged. We also now have the option of using a selection of clamps, penile sheaths and pads designed for modern living.

Urinary incontinence affects approximately 10 per cent of the male population. This number will always vary up and down depending on the questions men are asked. It remains a delicate and difficult subject to admit to. I see lots of women who tell me that they wish their husband would come to see me; sometimes they are persuaded and sometimes not, even if they know that their wife is having treatment and getting better.

You may have read or have heard problems with your urinary system referred to as LUTS; this just means lower urinary tract system. The *British Medical Journal* has found that over a third of men aged fifty are living with moderate to severe symptoms of LUTS. This equates to 3.4 million men in the UK and 24 million men in Europe. Please don't be one of them.

Stress Incontinence

This is something that often happens following a radical prostatectomy (see page 143) to treat prostate cancer.

It can also happen after a TURP (transurethral resection of the prostate) or laser prostatectomy. Both are performed to treat benign disease of your prostate. The aim is to improve the flow of urine if your prostate gland has grown too big and is obstructing the outflow of your urine. About 2 per cent of men suffer with a degree of incontinence following these procedures and this is usually stress incontinence. The answer in most cases is pelvic floor exercises.

Constipation and straining on the toilet, being overweight and excessive coughing can also be contributing factors, all made worse if you are a post-operative patient. So if you are about to have a radical prostatectomy or a TURP and you are struggling with your weight, constipation or a cough (maybe due to smoking), now is very definitely the time to take yourself in hand and do something about these issues.

Urge Incontinence

This can be caused by prostate surgery or it may happen quite out of the blue. It can happen if you are stressed, worrying about your job or your relationship. It could be caused by an excessive amount of caffeine, fizzy drinks or alcohol. Sometimes it is related to medication that you may be taking or an illness that you have, Parkinson's disease, stroke and MS to name a few. This can be quite a bewildering problem and, sadly, people may be less than understanding. However, it is very curable so do look at the advice in Chapter 4.

I hope the following story will make you feel less alone: a patient of mine who works in a high-stress and extremely busy environment came to see me in despair. He had been online and scared himself half to death reading things that had nothing to do with his problem. He had wet his bed as a child until he was about fourteen years old. His bladder had behaved itself reasonably well since then, although he went to the toilet about once an hour so that he was known among his friends as TB (tiny bladder)! However, the problem was manageable and he certainly was not having any incontinence. After university he had gone to work in a busy office where there were lots of long meetings and lots of coffee. His problems started to become much worse and the more he worried about it the worse it got. He was now occasionally not making it to the toilet in time and having a few accidents.

He had visited a urologist who had carried out all the tests to rule out any underlying problems, including a urodynamic study (this is a test to look at how well your bladder, urethra and sphincters are working; it also looks at what happens as your bladder fills and empties). They found that he had an overactive bladder. He started to take medication to try and calm his bladder down.

In a way he was hugely relieved to find the cause of his problem. He was then sent to see me and I taught him pelvic floor exercises and bladder training.

He was determined to get better and as a result he is now not having any accidents any more and has discontinued the pills.

Doing his pelvic floor exercises has given him the confidence to hold on until his meetings are over and bladder training means he has increased his bladder capacity so he is going less frequently. In addition, drinking less coffee was part of his plan and this seems to have helped too. His treatment has given him his life back.

Overflow Incontinence

Overflow incontinence can have the following symptoms:

- A poor urine stream or flow of urine
- Hesitancy to get the flow of urine started
- Having to push down on your pelvic floor muscles to try to pee. This often happens when your prostate gland is enlarged. This is something that you must deal with as it could lead to your bladder becoming overstretched and never working properly again

I have looked after lots of men who have ended up in A&E not being able to pass urine at all. Anyone who has been in this pickle will tell you that it is extremely painful. So the moral of this story is seek help before you end up like a patient of mine on a flight halfway to New York and in agony at not being able to pee.

Nocturia

This means that you have started to get up more than once in the night to pass urine. Getting up more frequently during the night to pass urine, particularly if you are over the age of fifty, is often the first sign of an enlarged prostate gland. If this is the case it's time to visit your doctor before your prostate gland grows any bigger. But there are other causes of nocturia. These may be an overactive bladder, an infection or possibly a period of anxiety in your life. It could also be caused by any drugs that you are taking, or an underlying medical condition like diabetes may be the problem. It could be something very simple like too much coffee or alcohol before bed. It may simply be a fact of ageing. Whatever the reason you need to find out why this is happening to you.

Nocturnal Enuresis

This is when you have started to wet the bed. This is serious and distressing. It could mean that you are not emptying your bladder properly or you have a urine infection – sometimes there doesn't seem to be a good explanation or it may be you are going through a stressful time in your life. Like nocturia, it may be that you just have a small or overactive bladder. It could be that you have been drinking too much alcohol or caffeinated drinks. Whatever the reason do seek medical help.

After Dribble

Post micturition dribble, after dribble – whatever you call it, it can leave an embarrassing wet patch on your underpants or, worse, on your trousers.

How many of you have been standing in the men's toilet and noticed the man next to you shaking and pulling his penis to try and extract the last drop of pee (even though you are trying hard not to look)? Maybe you have been doing this too?

It can happen to women but is much more common in men. It happens when your muscles do not close off tightly enough after passing urine and a little urine then leaks out. It can happen up to a few minutes after passing urine. As the male urethra is about 20cm long a little bit of urine pools in the urethra and slowly and passively trickles out as you move about.

This is a very irritating problem and definitely one that isn't discussed at dinner parties. How on earth do you make it go away?

I remember a patient who came to see me with this very problem. He had started by putting kitchen paper in his underpants but this just became damp and made his skin sore. So he had been using his girlfriend's sanitary towels cut in half and stuck in his underpants – not ideal, although he did say that it had made him much more aware of what women have to go through every month! He had been living like this for over two years. When I saw him I performed a bladder ultrasound scan to check he was emptying his bladder properly, and a urine test to check for infection. I started him on a regime of pelvic floor exercises and urethral milking (see below).

He also went on a diet, as he was considerably overweight. He is now better – the leakage has stopped and he is very pleased. He will keep doing his pelvic floor exercises every day, as he never wants the problem back. He has taken back control of his bladder. In this case it was not very clear what was the cause of his problem but excessive weight gain may well have been the reason.

Here are a few self-help tips for dealing with after dribble:

- Practise your pelvic floor exercises.
- Try sitting down to pass urine.
- Try urethral milking: place two fingers behind your testicles and try to milk the last drops of urine out of your urethra by pressing on your perineum and slowly moving your fingers upwards and forwards in a milking motion.
- Wear loose underpants or boxer shorts to avoid extra pressure on the perineum as this could force the urine out of the urethra and cause a leak.

The Prostate Gland

Recent research by the Urology Foundation found that two-thirds of the British public do not know what the prostate does.

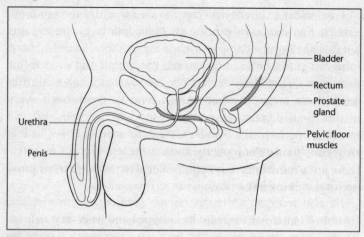

Prostate

The prostate is a small gland about the size of a walnut and is only found in men, women do not have one. It sits just below your bladder and in front of your rectum. Your urethra runs through it to allow urine to flow out from your bladder. The prostate secretes a fluid that helps to nourish your sperm and forms part of your semen, which comes out of your penis when you have an ejaculation. As you age sometimes your prostate gland grows bigger and can start to give you trouble.

We know that approximately 50 per cent of men in their sixties and 80 per cent of men aged seventy to ninety have an enlarged prostate; that's an awful lot of you chaps out there. Not all of you will necessarily need to do anything about it – just be sensible and seek help if you start to have symptoms. These can include: passing small amounts of urine very frequently and with urgency; finding it takes ages to pee and the flow has reduced to a trickle; hesitancy to start the flow; getting up at night to pee more than once or more than you used to. You may find that you are straining to pass urine and never emptying your bladder and this can lead to urine infections. These are all signs that you need to visit your doctor and start some form of treatment. These symptoms could also be a sign of prostate cancer so you really need to go and be checked out.

You may be asked to complete something called the International Prostate Symptom Score (IPSS). This consists of a series of questions that can help you and your doctor see how severe your symptoms are and how best to help you.

Treatment for an Enlarged Prostate
There are a number of ways you can deal with an enlarged prostate, depending on the severity of your symptoms.

- There are drugs to shrink or relax your prostate and help the flow of urine
- Lifestyle changes such as drinking fewer fizzy drinks, avoiding caffeine and alcohol, particularly late in the evening
- Trying to double void (see page 23)
- Sitting down to pee
- Avoiding constipation as this can really affect your urine flow
- Improve your diet and try to lose weight if you know you are overweight

Your doctor may decide with you to use these techniques with or without medication; this is often called watchful waiting, meaning the doctor will keep an eye on you. If things haven't improved, surgery can be performed, but only as a last resort.

Transurethral Resection of the Prostate (TURP)
This operation is performed for a benign enlarged prostate gland. It is usually done only after conservative measures (see above) have been tried. It generally involves a short stay in hospital and in most cases a general anaesthetic. The surgery is performed via your penis. Your urologist then removes small pieces of your prostate, using a heated wire loop, that is stopping your urine from

flowing well. This procedure can also be performed using a laser. This is done in a similar way via your penis.

It is rarely performed in men under forty years old. It is much more common in the over-fifties; about 15,000 men a year have a TURP in the UK.

Don't be afraid to seek help. I say this as I have looked after a lot of men over the years who were scared of the possible side effects of a prostate resection, which can include retrograde ejaculation (meaning that when you have an orgasm the semen goes into your bladder instead of coming out of the end of your penis). They have sometimes been just scared or embarrassed to go to the doctor about their urinary problems.

In some of these cases the prostate has obstructed the outflow of urine so much that their bladder has grown bigger and bigger and is unable to empty itself. This sometimes means that even after surgery you are not able to empty your bladder as it has been too stretched for too long and you will need to use a catheter to empty out your urine. Anyone who is reading this and knows that they should have visited the doctor months ago better get there ASAP. If including this information here stops even one man from overstretching his bladder I will be very happy.

One of my patients suffered from stress incontinence following a laser treatment to reduce the size of his prostate. He wrote about his experiences and has kindly allowed me to use some of his words here:

'My prostate first made its presence felt during my mid-fifties, when "having a wee" suddenly ceased to be what it was. What had always been a powerful jet dwindled to a mere trickle and three or four effortful tries were needed before my bladder felt empty. Like most men when things go wrong below the belt, I was overcome with squeamish embarrassment and told no one.'

He ended up having the laser procedure twice, first in 2005 and then again in 2012. It was after the second operation that his troubles started.

'Having not experienced incontinence after the earlier surgery, it was the last thing I expected. What I had was stress incontinence. As long as I sat or lay without moving, I was fine, but any kind of exertion or anxiety set it off.'

Five months later he found me and he started to improve with pelvic floor rehabilitation.

He says, 'Female stress incontinence is discussed quite openly, even with jolly little TV ads, but nothing is ever said about the male version.'

I hope that any of you who are reading this and struggling with symptoms realize that you are not alone. Do start by following the self-help advice above and I hope that it will give you the courage to seek the help that has made you read my book in the first place.

Radical Prostatectomy

A radical prostatectomy is performed if you have prostate cancer. It is an operation to remove your whole prostate and it can be performed in an open procedure (an incision in your stomach) or by keyhole surgery in the form of either laparoscopic or robotic surgery. This requires a hospital stay and a general anaesthetic as well as a period of recovery afterwards. You will recover more quickly if you have prepared yourself before the surgery by being as fit and healthy as you can be. Try to remember that this is a big operation so don't do too much too soon and listen to your body. If you are having lots of stress incontinence and wearing several pads a day, maybe you should not be playing golf or rushing off to the office – instead you should be resting a bit more.

There are studies to show that doing your pelvic floor exercises before radical prostate surgery is beneficial and certainly helps you in the first three months after your operation.[33] So if you are about to have a radical prostatectomy then you need to start a regime of exercises straight away. It will help you to understand where your muscles are and how they work before your operation. Afterwards you will be sore and generally recovering from the surgery. So if you already know how to do your pelvic floor exercises this will be a big help to you. You will be ahead of the curve. It is extremely important that you learn how to do the exercises and keep at them religiously.

Following radical prostatectomy you may have some urinary incontinence and erectile dysfunction. The type of incontinence that you usually have is stress incontinence (see page 30) and generally happens when you move about, so you will not wet the bed (lying down is fine). It also happens when you stand from a sitting position. Men tell me it often happens when they are bending down to dry their feet after a shower, which can be hugely frustrating. It can happen when you sneeze, cough, laugh or get out of your car or make a sudden movement. And it's often worse towards the end of the day when you are tired. It can also happen when you have an orgasm or are sexually stimulated, but don't be afraid if this happens to you.

I looked after a gentleman some years ago who had had a radical prostatectomy. I had seen him before his operation and taught him pelvic floor exercises; I then saw him after his surgery and he was dutifully doing his exercises. He was a fit, slim, energetic gentleman who had recently sold his business so he had lots of spare time on his hands. A few months later he came to see me in my clinic, feeling very sorry for himself. He was still wearing three pads a day and wanted to know what to do next.

We had a long chat about what he had been up to; he had taken to playing tennis four times a week with his friends. This would not have been so bad if he had been a worse tennis player. He was good, very good in fact, and as a result had been leaping about the court and delaying the recovery of his continence. He gave up tennis for a month, worked really hard on his pelvic floor exercises with some electrical stimulation as well, and about three months later he was better and dry and can now play tennis to his heart's content.

I have a patient who had had a robotic radical prostatectomy for prostate cancer four weeks before. He was in complete misery, wearing five pads a day and thinking this was the future. He was also very sore around his perineum and also in his groin. I explained to him that this could be quite normal at this early post-operative stage. In his bid to get better and return to his old life he had overworked his poor pelvic floor muscles.

With any robotic or laparoscopic surgery you physically recover much more quickly than if you have had open surgery (been cut open) for obvious reasons. The surgery is much less invasive. You heal quickly and feel well so it can be hard to understand why you are having stress incontinence, why every time you stand up from your chair you leak a bit of urine or, worse, if you go for a walk at the end of the day and end up damp. This is because your urethral sphincter is weak following the surgery.

The problem is you can't see your sphincter working as it's inside you. If the rest of your body has healed so well it's hard to understand why the inside is not working normally as well, although you were most likely told before the operation that this was one of the common side effects.

I explained all this to my patient and also explained that overdoing his pelvic floor exercises was not going to make him better more quickly. He therefore rested his muscles for two days, took to lying down for an hour after lunch, and then resumed his pelvic floor exercises following my instructions (see Chapter 2). He came back to see me four weeks later and he is now dry and delighted. He continues to wear a pad if he goes out at the moment but it is very much 'just in case'. I suspect he will soon be able to give this up.

I always advise patients who have undergone radical prostate surgery to carry on doing their pelvic floor exercises for life.

There are other treatments for prostate cancer, such as radiotherapy, hormone treatments and brachytherapy. Whatever treatment you are having it's a good idea to do your pelvic floor exercises as all of them can potentially cause urinary problems and erectile dysfunction.

Chronic Pelvic Pain Syndrome or Chronic Nonbacterial Prostatitis

I'd like to talk a little bit about this problem as the pelvic floor muscles can be used in a different way to ease the symptoms, instead focusing on releasing and relaxing the muscles.

The causes of chronic pelvic pain syndrome/chronic prostatitis are poorly understood. It may be caused by an infection or inflammation of the prostate gland. It is more commonly seen in younger men between thirty and fifty and is often difficult to treat. If it's any comfort to any of you who are suffering from the problem, it is not life-threatening although it can be debilitating and life-limiting. The symptoms you may have are pain or discomfort around your penis (often in the tip), testicles, anus or in your lower abdomen. There may be pain with peeing, a frequent or urgent need to pee, pain on ejaculation, pain after sexual intercourse and possibly erectile dysfunction.

There is no gold standard treatment for chronic pelvic pain but there are lots of things that you can do to help with the problems caused and the pain. You may need to see a urologist and antibiotics or other medications may help. It is also sometimes helpful to see a pain specialist.

Some self-help tips while you are waiting to see a specialist include:

- Take steps to avoid constipation as this can aggravate the problem (see Chapter 9).
- Try something called a reverse pelvic floor exercise, or reverse Kegels, to relax the pelvic floor, as normal pelvic floor exercises are not recommended. This is done by trying to relax the anal sphincter and imagine you are passing urine. Try doing this once a day and build up to three times per day. There is no exact amount of times

that you should carry this out so if it's helping do it regularly but stop if it is making things worse.

- You may find that acupuncture, herbal remedies and sometimes massage or hypnotherapy can help, but it's always best to check with your doctor before embarking on an alternative therapy just in case it might affect any treatment they have given you.

- You may find some benefit from counselling as chronic pain is a very hard thing to deal with. When you have a broken leg everyone gives you a huge amount of sympathy but chronic pain that only you are aware of is so much more difficult for people to understand and be sympathetic about. This makes it much more challenging to deal with. So please do seek help if you need someone to talk to.

Premature Ejaculation

This is a very important topic – see Chapter 8 for more information.

How to Cope with Ongoing Urinary Incontinence

There are a number of ways you can deal with the problems of urinary incontinence as a man.

Incontinence Pads

These are the first and easiest way of managing urine leakage. There are lots of different brands, shapes and sizes. They can be disposable or reusable so it is up to you as to which kind you would prefer to wear and which you would find the most comfortable. You can buy them in pharmacies, on the internet and even in the supermarket. You may be able to get them free from the NHS.

All too often I see men wearing women's pads. This is a terrible shame, as they don't fit the male anatomy or a man's underwear. Speaking of underpants, you will need to invest in fitted underpants, as boxer shorts will not really work to hold the pad in place. There are special thin pants made of a net-like material specially designed to hold the pads snugly in place. If you have these, you can then wear your boxer shorts on top of them. On the market there are male-shaped pads – they are a sort of triangular shape and come in various absorbencies. So if you have just the tiniest leak you can wear a thin little pad; with worse incontinence you can wear thicker and more absorbent pads. If your urine leakage is more severe there are ranges of pull-on pant-style pads that are much more absorbent and will keep you dry and safe.

Penile Clamps and Other Devices

There is also a selection of penile clamps on the market. I use one called Dribblestop. It is exactly as it says – a clamp for the penis. It fits behind the glans of the penis on the shaft. It is made of plastic and a type of foam that doesn't absorb liquid. The clamp only applies a slight pressure on the top and the bottom of the penis, so it doesn't restrict your blood circulation. You can therefore wear it all day if you wish; although you will need to release it every few hours to pass urine. It has different side pieces which make it fully adjustable to fit all varying sizes of penis and ensure a fit that is tight enough to stop urine leakage but not so tight as to be painful.

It works for both circumcised and uncircumcised men and can give you your freedom back, particularly if you are suffering from severe incontinence that one or two small pads will not cover. It means you can go and have a game of golf, go for a long walk, or whatever it is you fancy, without the worry of wet trousers.

The next group of products available are penile appliances of one type or another. In most cases you will need help at least on the first occasion with the correct fitting of the appliance. They include penile sheaths or condom catheters (they look very like a condom and are applied to the penis in the same way). These have an adhesive on the inside so when rolled on to the penis they stick and your urine drains into a small bag attached to your leg. The alternative is something called a body-worn urinal. They are usually held in place with straps or are integrated in a pair of underpants. In older gentlemen or obese men where the penis is shortened or retracted these devices will not work and pads are by far the best option.

Always remember, these products are there to help you in the short term – never see them as a permanent solution to your incontinence. In most cases and following prostate surgery they are there to help you keep your dignity and contain the problem while you are getting better.

Surgery

If you have severe stress incontinence for whatever reason surgery may become the best solution.

An artificial sphincter is a device that is implanted into your body under a general anaesthetic. It acts as your own sphincter once did to help keep you dry. It consists of three parts: a cuff that goes around your urethra; a pump that's put in your scrotum next to one of your testicles; and a reservoir of water that sits in your abdomen. It works by compression on your urethra. It is all internal so there is nothing to see on the outside of your body. When you feel the urge to pass urine, you go to the toilet and squeeze the pump in your scrotum; this opens the cuff and your urine can drain out. Over the next minute or two the cuff refills with water from the reservoir, again applying compression to your urethra, and you are dry once more.

You may also have a bulking agent injected into your bladder neck to try to keep your bladder neck closed and you dry.

Whatever you do, don't sit back and do nothing. So many of the treatments and devices we have discussed in this chapter can help or cure your problems. I hope that after reading this chapter you will start to pay more attention to your pelvic floor rehabilitation. Once you realize that not only is it simple to do but it can be life-changing and give you back your freedom, you will be energized to sort out all your pelvic floor dysfunction. Then both men and women together, and not just women alone, can start a pelvic floor revolution! Wouldn't that be fabulous!

GLOSSARY

An Explanation of a Few Commonly Performed Bladder and Bowel Tests

anal manometry: during this test a flexible tube is inserted into your rectum with a balloon attached. The balloon is inflated. Tests are then done to see how your rectum and anal sphincter are relaxing and contracting.

anal ultrasound: this test evaluates the structure of your anal sphincter with ultrasound images. A small probe is inserted into your anus while the test is being performed.

bladder scan or bladder ultrasound scan: this can be performed to check if your bladder is filling and emptying properly. It can also be used to look at the whole of your urinary tract (kidneys, ureters and bladder) to check for any problems.

colon transit study: a measurement of your colon transit, or how long food takes to pass through your bowel. You will be asked to swallow capsules containing small markers that show up on X-ray. After about five days you will have an X-ray to see if any or all of the markers have passed through. This will tell your doctor how quickly or slowly your bowels are working.

colonoscopy: this is when a thin flexible tube, known as a colonoscope, which has a light and a camera on the end, is passed through your anus. It is performed to examine the lining of your large bowel (intestine) for any problems.

cystogram: a study of your bladder, it is used to help diagnose any problems. Dye is inserted into your bladder using a catheter, following which X-rays are taken.

cystoscopy: a cystoscopy is when a thin telescope with a camera is passed up through your urethra (in women) or your penis (in men) to look inside and inspect your bladder. It also looks at your urethra and where your ureters enter your bladder. This procedure can be done with either a local or a general anaesthetic. The local anaesthetic version is often just to have a look inside your bladder and is done with something called a flexible cystoscope. The general anaesthetic version uses a bigger, rigid cystoscope and this is used if treatment to your bladder is needed.

defacating proctogram: this is a test to look at how your bowel and rectum look and work when you open your bowels. It looks at what happens to your pelvic floor in the act of bowel-opening. It is done either in an MRI (magnetic resonance imaging) scanner or with normal X-ray.

flow rate/test: you will be asked to have a full bladder and then pass urine through a machine called a flowmeter or uroflowmeter, which measures the speed of your urine flow and also the amount of urine that you have passed.

post-voided residual urine: you will first have a scan of your bladder while it is full, then you will be asked to go and empty it as best you can. A second bladder scan is performed to see if you bladder is now empty. If it is not and urine is left behind, this is called the post-voided residual volume of urine.

total pelvic floor ultrasound: this is an ultrasound scan to assess your pelvic floor function (women); you will be asked to do things like contracting and relaxing your pelvic floor, coughing and bearing down.

urine test (urinalysis): your urine can be tested in different ways either in the doctor's surgery by simple dipstick examination or your urine can be sent away to the laboratory to be examined in more detail under the microscope. Urinalysis can reveal a lot about our general health and is a simple and very useful tool for diagnosing things such as diabetes, kidney disease and urine infections. Urine tests also are often the first signs of pregnancy and therefore the bringer of very happy news.

urodynamics: a urodynamic test is done to assess bladder, urinary sphincter and urethral function. It is a test to see how everything is working, and it also looks at how we fill and empty our bladder.

HELPFUL ORGANIZATIONS

General Health and Wellbeing

ASH (Action on Smoking and Health) and **QUIT** support smokers to stop smoking.
www.ash.org.uk and www.quit.org.uk

The British Dietetic Association provides food factsheets to help you learn the best ways to eat and drink to keep your body fit and healthy.
www.bda.uk.com/foodfacts/home

Drinkaware works to reduce alcohol misuse and harm in the UK.
www.drinkaware.co.uk

www.embarrassingissues.co.uk
www.embarrassingproblems.com

HMSA (Hypermobility Syndromes Association) provides support for people with hypermobility-related disorders.
hypermobility.org

Mindfulness: A Practical Guide to Finding Peace in a Frantic World, by Mark Williams and Dr Danny Penman, Piatkus, 2011

NHS website has lots of advice, tips and tools to help you make the best choices about your health and wellbeing.
www.nhs.uk

Teenagers

ERIC (The Children's Bowel and Bladder Charity) is the only charity dedicated to the bowel and bladder health of all children and teenagers in the UK.
www.eric.org.uk

Great Ormond Street Hospital also has a pelvic floor exercise sheet for young people.
www.gosh.nhs.uk/teenagers/your-condition/tests-and-treatments/pelvic-floor-muscle-exercises

NHS Highland have produced a YouTube video especially for teenagers called *Your Pelvic Floor*.
www.youtube.com/watch?v=v731EXFR2k4

'Your Pelvic Floor' is an award-winning leaflet aimed at teenagers and is available online or from your local continence clinic.

Pelvic Floor Exercises

Elvie is an award-winning pelvic floor trainer that uses biofeedback to help you track your progress.
www.elvie.com

Squeezy is an award-winning app produced by the NHS. Now there is one for men as well.
www.squeezyapp.com

Pregnancy

The American College of Obstetricians and Gynecologists have a website with lots of useful information for women.
www.acog.org

The MASIC Foundation (Mothers with Anal Sphincter Injuries in Childbirth) aims to reduce the incidence of birth injury, as well as helping new mothers who may be suffering in silence from its symptoms, which are all too often hidden in society.
masic.org.uk

Mumsnet ('by parents for parents') makes parents' lives easier by pooling knowledge, advice and support on everything from conception to childbirth, from babies to teenagers.
www.mumsnet.com

Pelvic, Obstetric and Gynaecological Physiotherapy (POGP) have lots of useful information leaflets.
www.pogp.csp.org.uk

The Royal College of Midwives
www.rcm.org.uk

The Royal College of Obstetricians and Gynaecologists have a section on their website containing a range of resources designed for women and the public.
www.rcog.org.uk

Wellbeing of Women is a charity dedicated to improving the health of women and their babies.
www.wellbeingofwomen.org.uk

Menopause

The Daisy Network is dedicated to providing information and support to women diagnosed with premature ovarian insufficiency, also known as premature menopause.
www.daisynetwork.org.uk

International Menopause Society – the aims of the IMS are to promote knowledge, study and research on all aspects of ageing in women.
www.imsociety.org

The Menopause Exchange gives advice about the menopause, midlife and postmenopausal health.
www.menopause-exchange.co.uk

North American Menopause Society – focused on the menopause, NAMS provides physicians, practitioners and women with essential menopause information.
www.menopause.org

Women's Health Concern is the patient arm of the British Menopause Society.
www.womens-health-concern.org

Sex

The British Society for the Study of Vulval Diseases is a medical organization and has clinics around the country.
https://bssvd.org

The Sexual Advice Association is a charitable organization created to help improve the sexual health and wellbeing of men and women. They have also produced the SMART SAA app to provide reliable, confidential sexual health advice to men and women.
sexualadviceassociation.co.uk

The Vulval Pain Society promotes and protects the physical and mental health of sufferers of vulval pain through the provision of support, education and practical advice.
www.vulvalpainsociety.org

Bowel Problems

Bowel Disease Research Foundation
www.bdrf.org.uk

British Society of Gastroenterology – their website has lots of patient resources relating to gastroenterology.
www.bsg.org.uk

Crohn's and Colitis UK is the UK's leading charity in the battle against Crohn's disease and ulcerative colitis.
www.crohnsandcolitis.org.uk

Guts UK is committed to fighting all digestive disorders.
gutscharity.org.uk

The IBS Network is the UK's national charity for IBS, offering information, advice and support for patients with IBS.
www.theibsnetwork.org

Men

Manversation is a campaign focused on encouraging men with advanced prostate cancer to have conversations with their healthcare team.
www.manversation.co.uk

Men's Health Forum is a British registered charity whose mission is to improve the health of men and boys in England, Wales and Scotland.
www.menshealthforum.org.uk

Orchid is a charity supporting men affected by male (prostate, testicular and penile) cancer.
orchid-cancer.org.uk

TrueNTH is a global initiative led by the Movember Foundation, tackling critical areas of prostate cancer care and helping men with their journey through prostate cancer.
us.truenth.org

Urinary Urgency, Frequency and Incontinence

Association for Continence Advice
www.aca.uk.com

The Bladder and Bowel Community helps support the millions of people in the UK who are living with conditions that affect the

bladder and bowel. Contact them to get hold of a 'Just Can't Wait' card (or download the app).
Tel: 01926 357220
www.bladderandbowel.org

Bladder Health UK (formerly known as the Cystitis and Overactive Bladder Foundation) gives support to people with all forms of cystitis, overactive bladder and continence issues, and their family and friends.
Tel: 0121 702 0820
bladderhealthuk.org

The British Association of Urological Nurses has a website that provides reliable information for patients on urological diseases that is unbiased, comprehensive and clear.
www.baun.co.uk/patients/

The British Association of Urological Surgeons (BAUS) has patient information on their website about all things to do with urology: your kidneys, bladder, prostate, including incontinence, impotence, infertility, cancer and reconstruction of the genito-urinary tract.
www.baus.org.uk

Continence Product Advisor is a worldwide organization helping people to manage their incontinence.
www.continenceproductadvisor.org

The European Association of Urology (EAU) aims to raise the level of urological care in Europe. It has trustworthy and up-to-date information for patients.
www.uroweb.org

The Great British Public Toilet Map is the UK's largest database of publicly accessible toilets.
www.toiletmap.org.uk

The International Continence Society
www.ics.org

The Simon Foundation for Continence is dedicated to bringing the topic of incontinence out into the open and providing help and hope for people with incontinence, their families and the healthcare professionals who provide their care.
simonfoundation.org

The Urology Foundation
Tel: 020 7713 9538
www.theurologyfoundation.org

REFERENCES

1 'Urinary incontinence in female athletes: a systemic review'; de Mattos Lourenco, T. R., Matsuoka, P. K., Baracat, E. C. and Haddad, J. M. *International Urogynecology Journal*, Dec. 2018; 29(12) pp. 1,757–63

2 'Progressive resistance exercise in the functional restoration of the perineal muscles'; Dumoulin, C., Cacciari, L. P. and Hay-Smith, E. J. C. *Cochrane Database of Systematic Reviews*, 4 October 2018

3 'Progressive resistance exercise in the functional restoration of the perineal muscles'; Arnold H. Kegel, MD, FACS, *American Journal of Obstetrics and Gynecology*, Aug. 1948; 56(2) pp. 238–48

4 'A group based yoga therapy intervention for urinary incontinence in women: a pilot randomized trial'; Huang, A. J., Jenny, H. E., Chesney, M. A., Schembri, M. and Subak, L. L. *Female Pelvic Medicine and Reconstructive Surgery*, May–June 2014; 20(3) pp. 147–54

5 'A randomized clinical trial comparing pelvic floor muscle training to a Pilates exercise program for improving pelvic muscle strength'; Culligan, P. J., Scherer, J., Dyer, K., Priestley, J. L., Guingon-White, G., Delveccio, D. and Vangeli, M. *International Urogynecology Journal*, 21 April 2010; 21(4) pp. 401–8

6 'Non-invasive electrical stimulation for stress incontinence in women'; Stewart, F., Berghmans, B., Bo, K. and Glazener, C. M. A. *Cochrane Database of Systematic Reviews*, 22 December 2017

7 'Stress Urinary Incontinence in Female Athletes'; Heath, A., Folan, S., Ripa, B., Varriale, C., Bowers, A., Gwyer, J. and Figuers, C. *Journal of Women's Health Physical Therapy*, Sep.–Dec. 2014; vol. 38(3), pp. 104–7

8 'Physiotherapy for women with stress urinary incontinence: a review article'; Ghaderi, F. and Oskouei, A. E. *Journal of Physical Therapy Science*, Sep. 2014

9 'Sustained therapeutic effects of percutaneous tibial nerve stimulation: 2-month results of the STEP study'; Peters, K. M., Carrico, D. J., MacDiarmid, S. A. et al. *Neurourology and Urodynamics*, Jan. 2013; 32(1) pp 24–9

10 'The history of pelvic organ prolapse from antiquity to present day'; Mattimore, J., Cheetham, P. and Katz, A. *Journal of Urology*, April 2015; vol. 193 (4)

11 'Uterine prolapse: from antiquity to today'; Downing, K. T. *Obstetrics and Gynecology International*, vol. 2012, Article ID 649459, 9 pages

12 'Understanding weight gain at menopause'; Davis, S. R., Castelo-Branco, C., Chedraui, P., Lumsden, M. A., Nappi, R. E., Shah, D. and Villaseca, P. as the writing group of the International Menopause Society for World Menopause Day 2012. *Climacteric* 2012, Oct.; 15(5) pp. 419–29

13 'Prolapse and sexual function in women with benign joint hypermobility syndrome'; Mastoroudes, H., Giarenis, I., Cardozo, L., Srikrishna, S., Vella, M., Robinson, D., Kazkar, H. and Grahame, R. *An International Journal of Obstetrics and Gynaecology*, Jan. 2013; 120(2) pp. 187–92

14 'Pelvic floor muscle training during pregnancy to prevent urinary incontinence: a single-blind randomized controlled trial'; Morkved, S., Bo, K., Schei, B. and Salvesen, K. A. *Obstetrics and Gynecology*, Feb. 2003; 101(2) pp. 313-19

15 'Pelvic floor muscle training for prevention and treatment of urinary and faecal incontinence in antenatal and postnatal women'; Woodley, S. J., Boyle, R., Cody, J. D., Morkved, S. and Hay-Smith, E. J. C. *Cochrane Database of Systematic Reviews*, Dec. 2017

16 'Interventions for treating constipation in pregnancy'; Jewell, D. J. and Young, G. *Cochrane Database of Systematic Reviews*, 2001

17 'Perineal assessment and repair longitudinal study (PEARLS): protocol for a matched pair cluster trial'; Bick, D. E., Kettle, C., Macdonald S., Thomas, P. W., Hills, R. K. and Ismail, K. M. *BMC Pregnancy and Childbirth*, 25 Feb. 2010

18 'Antenatal perineal massage for reducing perineal trauma'; Beckmann, M. M. and Stock, O. M. *Cochrane Database of Systematic Reviews*, April 2013

19 'Women's sexual health after childbirth'; Barrett, G., Pendry, E., Peacock, J., Victor, C., Thaker, R. and Manyonda, I. *British Journal of Obstetrics and Gynaecology*, Feb. 2000; 107(2) pp. 186–95

20 'Women's experience of menopause: a systemic review of qualitative evidence'; Hoga, L., Rodolpho, J., Goncalves, B. and Quirino, B. *JBI Database System Review*, Sep. 2015

21 'Urinary tract infections in postmenopausal women'; Raz, R. *Korean Journal of Urology*, Dec. 2011; 52(12) pp. 801–8

22 'Understanding weight gain at menopause'; Davis, S. R., Castelo-Branco, C., Chedraui, P., Lumsden, M. A., Nappi, R. E., Shah, D. and Villaseca, P. as the writing group of the International Menopause Society for World Menopause Day 2012. *Climacteric* 2012

23 ibid.

24 'Acupuncture in menopause (AIM) study: a pragmatic, randomized controlled trial'; Avis, N. E., Coeytaux, R. R., Isom, S., Prevette, K. and Morgan, T. *Menopause*, June 2016; 23(6) pp. 626–37

25 'National survey of sexual attitudes and lifestyles (Natsal-3)'; carried out by the London School of Hygiene and Tropical Medicine, University College London and NatCen Social Research

26 'Postpartum sexual function of women and the effects of early pelvic floor muscle exercises'; Citak, N., Cam, C., Arslan, H., Karateke, A., Tug, N., Ayaz, R. and Celik, C. *Acta Obstetrica et Gynecologica Scandinavica*, June 2010; 89(6) pp. 817–22

27 British Association of Dermatologists patient information leaflet on vulvodynia

28 'Rate and related factors of dyspareunia in reproductive age women: a cross-sectional study'; Sobhgol, S. S. and Alizadeli Charndabee, S. M. *International Journal of Impotence Research*, Jan.–Feb. 2007; 19(1) pp. 88–94

29 'Current therapies for premature ejaculation'; Gurs, S., Kadowitz, P. J. and Sikka, S.C. *Drug Discovery Today*, July 2016; 21(7) pp. 1,147–54

30 Adapted from 'Development of an abridged, 5-item version of the International Index of Erectile Function (IIEF-5) as a diagnostic tool for erectile dysfunction'; Rosen, R. C., Cappelleri, J. C., Smith, M. D., Lipsky, J. and Peña, B. M. *International Journal of Impotence Research*, Dec. 1999; 11(6) pp. 319–26

31 'Controversies and recent developments of the low-FODMAP diet'; Hill, P., Muir, J. G. and Gibson, P. R. *Gastroenterology and Hepatology*, Jan. 2017; 13(1) pp. 36–45

32 'The leaky faucet: a history of the treatment of male urinary incontinence'; Chong, J. and Simma-Chiang, V. *Journal of Urology*, May 2017; vol. 197, p. 1,063

33 'Preoperative pelvic floor muscles exercise and postprostatectomy incontinence: a systemic review and meta-analysis'; Chang, J. I., Lam, V. and Patel, M. *Journal of European Urology*, March 2016; 69(3) pp. 460–67

ACKNOWLEDGEMENTS

Firstly, to all my patients, without whom there would not be a book at all. You have all been so strong and brave in facing difficult, personal and often embarrassing problems with truly humbling courage. Thank you.

To my husband, William, and to my stepson, Charles, who are the lights of my life. Thank you both for your love and always being there for me. None of this would have been possible without you two. Also, thank you for putting up with me, and with rather more ready meals than normal during the writing process!

To my wonderful family who have made me who I am today and who I adore with all my heart: to my mother and brother, Richard, and in the memory of my father, Peter, who I think would have just said 'marvellous' that his daughter had written a book – we all miss him very much.

To the rest of my family: Anna, Marcus, Caleb, Amelia, Edward, Muriel, Caroline, Ed and Isobel; you are the best, I love you all very much.

To Anna Van Trigt, my amazing PA, and to the fab Megan Clewes, who puts up with me every day and has kept me sane during the writing of my book!

To Georgia Coleridge who pushed me to write the book in the first place. Thank you, Georgia.

To Caroline Michel and everyone at Peters Fraser and Dunlop, including Tim Binding, Laurie Robertson and Lucy Irvine; thank you all so much for having faith in me.

To the Penguin team: firstly, my editor, Martina O'Sullivan, thank you for all your help and patience with me as a brand-new author; and to Celia Buzuk, Julia Murday, Josie Murdoch, Clare Sayer, Elisabeth Merriman, Pat Rush, Rachael Tremlett and Ellie Smith, and to everyone else on the team who has worked so hard to make this whole thing happen.

To all my wonderful medical colleagues who work away tirelessly every day treating patients and helping them to have the best quality of life possible.

To my very good friends Jayne and Anthony, Tarek and Susie, and Clare and Richard, who have always been there for me.

INDEX